Fascia

A Science-based Guide to Reducing
Joint Pain

*(The Science and Clinical Applications in Manual
and Movement Therapy)*

Marvin Lacroix

Published By **Ryan Princeton**

Marvin Lacroix

All Rights Reserved

Fascia: A Science-based Guide to Reducing Joint Pain (The Science and Clinical Applications in Manual and Movement Therapy)

ISBN 978-1-998038-01-5

No part of this guidebook shall be reproduced in any form without permission in writing from the publisher except in the case of brief quotations embodied in critical articles or reviews.

Legal & Disclaimer

Table Of Contents

Chapter 1: On Fascia

1. What is fascia?

Fascia is tissue that anatomists used to carelessly reduce apart and throw away. Some of it's miles moist, cobweb-like tissue that lies among or on top of the systems being tested. In a steak, the ones whitish structures are honestly seen within the pink muscle groups. It is most effective for the motive that first Fascia Research Congress in 2007 on the Harvard Medical School that medication's courting to this apparently stupid filler material has modified dramatically.

Fascia, additionally called connective tissue, is positioned everywhere in the body. It is what gives our organs, blood vessels, muscle tissues and tremendous frame tissues their shape. Fascia seamlessly flows into every one in every of a kind, and can each transmit and take in anxiety. This is the way it connects the whole thing in our frame to the whole thing else – and as it connects all systems in the frame, it is the missing hyperlink that lets in holistic, conventional treatments to be understood from a systematic aspect of view.

Fascia is densely full of sensory nerves that transmit records approximately the frame's characteristic in region and which may be moreover capable of signal ache.

As we realise, our body is basically crafted from fluids. Fluid is placed not only inside the cells, but also around them. This fluid is also called lymph. It is vital for the fascia to paintings nicely. If the fascia isn't sufficiently stimulated via motion, strain and traction, it will become sticky due to the truth the fluid, which incorporates adhesive proteins, isn't moved spherical well. Such raveled and sticky fascia is greater sensitive to stimuli of ache and the frame loses flexibility and resilience.

But such adhesions of the fascia can be launched over again and the frame can regain its elasticity and power thru fascial schooling.

2. How can fascia gain expertise of?

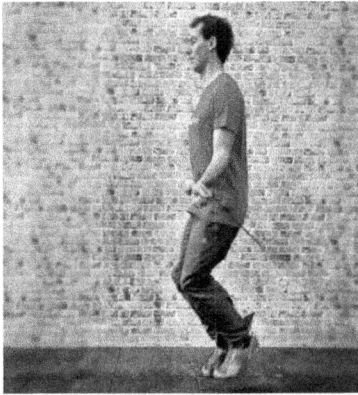

Like almost all tissue inside the frame, fascia is in a constant way of model to its environment and the frame's performance necessities. Fascia can contribute to stability, mobility and versatility. It responds to external stimuli. These stimuli reason the exceptional fascial tissues to tighten, to slip on pinnacle of each special or to intertwine. This continues the lymphatic fluid in amongst transferring as well, like a lubricant, and the fasciae do no longer stick together.

The best fascial education may additionally need to take whole advantage of the whole kind of movement of the body. Fascia loves 3-dimensional, free-flowing movements, which includes the ones finished in dance or in some martial arts.

3

3. Why Qi Gong is good for fascial schooling

Qi Gong is a top notch way to go into the arena of holistic training as it combines very gradual, flowing actions with mindfulness and breathwork and within reason smooth to test. Qi Gong is each a factor of diverse martial arts and a pillar of Traditional Chinese Medicine. This shape of exercise for health has been delicate over lots of years and way to fascia research, we are now able to understand how and why it truly works in a holistic manner.

Generally, any sort of motion stimulates the fascia. Walking, for instance, consists of a huge amount of fasciae, thinking about that this movement stretches from the ft to at least the shoulders. Sitting in an place of business chair and shifting simplest the palms at the keyboard correspondingly trains fewer fasciae. The spine specifically is generally not sufficiently exercised. The spine is an extremely mobile form. Therefore, people working with fascia like to seek advice from it because the 'vertebral snake'. If mobility isn't always exercised, the fascia throughout the spine turns into disheveled and sticks together over time. It then turns into increasingly more of a pole, held stable and tight in the function in which it's miles used most of the day.

Holistic exercise programs bear in mind this loss of activity of the backbone and sell its flexibility. In Qi Gong there are actions regarding ahead folds and backbends, rotations and sidebends. Even all through although or popularity Qi Gong, in which there can be every so often any movement, the backbone movements lightly with the breath, even greater in order the respiratory becomes greater natural and cushty. The spine stretches barely at some point of inhalation – throughout exhalation it barely collapses and the pinnacle frame tilts ahead. Through mindfulness in silence, practising Qi Gong moreover permits to grow to be aware about any anxiety and to release it from the interior out. The a first-rate deal much less tension there is in the frame and specially across the backbone, the less hard it's miles to respire – and the extra fluently power can bypass via the fasciae alongside the functional channels, moreover known as meridians, in the body.

Functional channels are chains of muscle tissues that co-characteristic to perform an motion. These muscle chains are related via fascia and can transmit both pressure and anxiety. If those muscle chains do not art work together in the awesome feasible way, man or woman muscle mass want to paintings more difficult and this may result in a pressure inside the corresponding place. In Traditional Chinese Medicine (TCM), as in physiotherapy, that is referred to as a blockage. TCM states that the go together with the flow of power is impaired, even as in physiotherapy this has a tendency to consult joints that now not follow the go together with the waft of movement. What every structures have in common is that the connection in the go along with the flow of motion need to be restored if you need to gather regular mobility. The techniques used are also very similar in each structures. Ideally, they ensure unrestricted mobility and the unobstructed transmission of pressure in the fascial muscle chains/meridians.

three.1 Fascial schooling inspired through nature

Fascial education as a end result pastimes at making the frame as comfortable and effective as viable. It is the form of relaxed state that animals have at the same time as we've a study them within the wild. But it could moreover be seen in our tom cat and dog pets. When you stroke them, you may enjoy their softness and understand their moderate actions, no matter the reality that they also can exert an entire lot of pressure in assessment to their body duration. When the fascia is clean and supple, the transmission of pressure and execution of motion can take area at an top of the line degree. With growing age or lack of exercise, people gather increasingly more blockages until movement becomes tough and lacks smoothness. By operating in the direction of Qi Gong, this suppleness of movements may be preserved. "Pliant like a bamboo, robust like a lumberjack," says an vintage proverb, for instance. This is why the physical sports are achieved slowly, just so there can be time to be gift with interest constantly and to have a look at the body on the equal time as acting the movements, which allows to stumble on and launch anxiety. As a result, those moves usually appearance mild and playful.

This principle of softness can be discovered particularly properly in expert acrobats. They regularly outwardly appear very slim and but are able to splendid feats, collectively with repute in a one-arm handstand or effortlessly pulling themselves up a rope. These are talents that well-educated guys with visibly stated muscle corporations aren't often able to. What subjects in the ones varieties of movements is not the diameter of person muscle groups, however the clean interplay of the sensible chains – in different phrases, the relaxation functionality of the entire muscle chains which may be required to paintings collectively. If there may be a blockage someplace within the respective useful channel, strengthening the muscle mass within the preference of enhancing motion is often of little use if it is not taken under attention how the muscle mass engage. When blockades are launched, the interplay between the muscle mass and the tissue is superior and mobility will growth.

three.2 Problems related to blockages at some stage in motion and fascial training

This interaction may be 'blocked' for numerous reasons, i.E. It does not work properly. When reading a brand new movement, for instance, the right interaction, the coordination of the sequences need to first be bodily understood. This can make the effort, counting on the complexity of the movement possibly even years. During physical mastering, outstanding sensible chains are activated, experimenting with wonderful tensions until the proper is placed. Once a motion has been mastered, most effective no less than anxiety is needed to perform it. The body then uses all its available sources to make the movement as green and easy as feasible. At that element, we no longer regularly need to concentrate on the execution of the mission. Everyone has skilled this even as the usage of a car: Initially, learning to shift gears have turn out to be tedious, but later you don't even need to think approximately it.

Type of blockage

Manifests in

Influencing factors

anxiety

bloodless sensation

attitude

alignment

warmth sensation

situation

weak point

noises in the joints

exercising behavior

reputation

ache

capability to pay attention

The desk above offers a quick assessment of various blockages. I in my opinion like to differentiate generally among weak point and anxiety. A mixture of vulnerable point and anxiety - which may be very not unusual - leads to misalignment. That manner that the alignment of the frame and specially the posture and function of the joints are not best for physical hobby. Feeling 'blocked' is frequently related to tension that has been present over an prolonged time body. Or because of a loss of motion in children the precise hobby and manage has no longer even been advanced for fine motion styles.

How those blockages display up can be very exquisite for everybody. The table shows the sensations that I determined maximum frequently. With anxiety, the corresponding place usually feels each bloodless or warmness. It is normally warmness at the begin and then, due to the fact the anxiety persists, cold in a while. If the body is placed underneath pressure in bad alignment, it can with out issues come to be strained, fundamental to contamination, which regularly manifests as warmth. In instances of inclined issue, there can be frequently noise at some point of motion. The joints start to crack. The lack of awareness, which frequently is going hand in hand with anxiety, and not using a trouble manifests in pain to make itself acknowledged.

three.Three Mindfulness and self-consciousness

Chapter 2: In Fascial Schooling

If hobby in one location isn't always well advanced or has been misplaced, it is able to be re-acquired via manner of interest and mindfulness. It is probably that here's a information of being overwhelmed in severa areas of life which has avoided the man or woman from having the ability draw their interest to their physical self every so often. Here I truly mean moments in which we loosen up and in quick turn our reputation to ourselves, with out being distracted with the useful resource of an excessive amount of of the outside global.

Weakness frequently is a stop end end result of terrible exercising behavior, which - like horrible contrary numbers to e.G. Brushing ones teeth - are created as a dependancy in the course of children. Just as we want great food to nourish the body in a wholesome and balanced way, we moreover want precise styles of exercise for our frame to be energetic.

Tension is regularly fuelled through way of our mind-set and attitudes. How masses importance I hook up with a few detail someone says is based upon on my individual mind-set. If a few factor weighs closely on me or if I want to collect some thing the least bit charges, this necessarily ends in tension in the frame.

This moreover explains why alignment, this is, my feature in location, may be specific relying at the situation. Based on my thoughts-set and attitude, effective conditions result in tensions in my body, which in flip exchange my posture and as a end result have an impact on my alignment. Situations can consequently - depending by myself evaluation - absolutely have a electricity on how I bodily pass thru a scenario.

four. The five requirements of fascial education

The bodily video games ought to to cover one or extra of those thoughts. The greater of them which is probably protected, the better. Put in adjectives, the five concepts are:

•3-dimensional

•bouncy/swinging/rhythmic

•aware

•flowing

•slowly and speedy

four.1 Why three-dimensional movements?

The connective tissue in our body is designed to face as a whole lot as the wishes of normal existence and then some. These normal sports, which vary substantially from man or woman to character, generate the stimuli the tissue wishes to come to be flawlessly aligned with the direction of hysteria or compression. These forces, affecting our our our bodies due to our sports, are rarely geared in the course of the correct alignment of person muscle mass or joints, however as an opportunity effect our ligaments, joints and muscle businesses from every capability direction and mind-set. For example, if electricity training is only ever practiced in a unmarried unique axis, the body could be sturdy for the duration of this exercising but beaten at the same time as energy needs to be implemented from a one in all a type mindset, as is often the case in normal existence. For instance, on the equal time as bending and lifting objects, cleansing and tidying, and playing, maximum humans bend, tilt, and twist through one-of-a-kind planes at the same time. The frame is designed to carry out the task to hand, no longer to transport stiffly via location on one plane.

If the body is robotically furnished with obligations in which this mobility may be finished, then it's miles going to be maintained along aspect the assisting muscular tissues, ligaments and fascial systems. Depending at the requirements, fascia can also offer extra balance or greater elasticity. The tissue adapts to the needs being made on a ordinary foundation. Ideally, the tissue is resilient in all three dimensions, which may be done thru suitable schooling that completely exhausts the frame's entire range of movement and skills.

Bone tissue behaves in exactly the identical manner, with the beneficial aid of the way. Depending on the direction of the loading purpose, the first-class bone bellows, which make a bone moderate and strong, align themselves on this form of manner that the bone turns into mainly resilient in the course of the load and on the equal time continues a positive simple balance.

The fascinating component is that the frame looks after itself and constantly has a hint extra balance and mobility in reserve than it desires in normal life. This reduces the probability of overuse injuries. Sportspeople are acquainted with this phenomenon referred to as supercompensation.

4.2 Why bouncy, swinging and rhythmic?

Soft fascia loves mild, swinging, rhythmic moves. In truth, the exact opposite of the inflexible postures we are subjected to in our each day work or school lives. These rhythmic, bouncy moves compress and squeeze the fascia like a sponge, and they amplify over again whilst they may be launched. Other fascia, which underneath tension stretches in commands, behaves like an elastic band, a rubber wire, this is pulled aside and then rhythmically returns to its relaxed u . S .. Also the pulling apart results in a 'squeezing out' of the fluid within the fibres of the fasciae, which right away remoisten at the same time as the tension is launched. In this way, the fascia is optimally furnished with nutrients. Water is very essential for the fascia: inflexible postures, repetitive moves and one-sided pressure reason the fascia to lose moisture and some of its capability. Simple actions then begin to turn out to be strenuous, they appearance jerky and awkward. It is tough to expect a healthful animal being capable of circulate efficaciously in nature with a stiff backbone. What could probable the gait of a canine or cat look like if the backbone had emerge as stiff and immobile? In order to permit the most variety of motion, the 24 vertebrae of the spinal column are generally no longer firmly fused together. However, if the backbone is stored inflexible maximum of the time, the fascial tissue for the duration of the movable vertebrae is the primary element to grow to be matted and glued collectively. Later, this can additionally result in abnormalities inside the joints. If the spine is commonly stored upright, it becomes immobile however nevertheless stays upright. This is of direction higher than inflexible and crooked – but it is even better to preserve the 'vertebral snake' cell. This additionally has blessings for the mobility of the legs and arms and the transmission of forces through the fascial connections (meridians) from the legs to the fingers and vice versa.

Dancing is surely one of the oldest styles of workout for human beings. In loose dance, we intuitively pass in all instructions and swing with our whole frame. This regularly creates a totally brilliant feeling of warmth and relaxation, openness and strength. The maximum critical difficulty is that we pass considerably and feel our entire body. The rhythmic bouncing traumatic conditions the fasciae and relaxes the muscle groups. In this way, mobility and power can be restored in a natural manner.

In remarkable phrases, fascia wishes slight bouncing and rhythmic movements to preserve its elasticity.

4.Three Why conscious?

Especially under the pores and pores and pores and skin, the fascia is complete of sensory cells.

Mindfulness can consequently in addition increase the stimulation of the fascia. With multiplied awareness, the sensory cells are inspired to accumulate more statistics. This effects in better blood move inside the vicinity and as a result to greater rest in the long time.

Intensified cognition also outcomes in a extra sensitive and unique coordination of the sequences of movements. Muscle hobby is more finely tuned and, if feasible, distributed over the complete body. Overall, mindful moves are commonly greater supple and relaxed. As a stop end result, the body relaxes inside the direction of the exercise and the movement. Here, the fascia plays an essential characteristic, because it lets in the frame to transmit strain over individual muscle groups. Furthermore, it could save and release kinetic strength in bouncing movements. This works terrific even as the muscular tissues do now not hinder this technique with tightness. Anxiety, as an example, can reason muscle tissues to emerge as chronically tight. For new movements, it regularly takes many hours of exercise with complete focus, for the muscle coordination to run easily, for vain anxiety to be released at a few level within the motion, and for the entire motion to be achieved results and with out a number of attention.

Mindfulness will growth the effectiveness of any fascial training. Even movements to which we usually do no longer pay unique interest, consisting of taking walks, can end up more supple. In the course of life, it frequently takes place that pointless tensions creep into movement styles after which become a dependancy. In the long term, the ones masses plenty much less than nice conduct can bring about troubles. Because of the reality that the weight on character structures is simply too immoderate and isn't always nicely allotted amongst severa systems, the muscle tissues, tendons or joints placed on out or end up infected more with out problem. Regular mindfulness training serves as a safety degree. Mindfulness improves the conscious perception of hysteria and allows rest. Walking meditation, as an instance, is brilliant for making on foot smoother and as a stop end result lowering shocks to the joints because of 'hard' strolling.

21

In walking meditation, each step is taken as consciously as feasible in sluggish motion and the focal point is at the weight shift in each step. This offers the cerebellum the possibility to re-coordinate already saved motion sequences and to optimize the movement collection. Movements in Qi Gong and Tai Chi are similar. They are carried out slowly and repeated regularly, so that the body has time to find out the perfect and maximum comfortable manner to perform the given movement. This takes location extra or less routinely, that's why traditional training in those movement arts encourages the scholar to exercise the shape - i.E. A exceptional collection of actions - over and over all over again. The greater a motion is repeated, the better it could be explored in all its detail, together with its relation to the relaxation of the body.

Fascia adapts to how the body is used and the frame plays what the mind requests. In the method, we draw on located skills and 'programs'. These movement packages need to moreover be refreshed from time to time to conform to modifications and current situations. If we neglect approximately those 'updates', how actions are completed often will become sloppy and disrupted by way of tightness. The fascial lines of traction work together an entire lot less correctly and the fascial tissue in substantial loses tone and elasticity as it is a whole lot much less worried in transmitting strain. If we forget about the sensations in our body for too prolonged, the 'purchaser' can be reminded of their frame via pain. How else is the body alleged to speak the urgency of its desires to our cerebrum? Pain automatically draws the attention back to the frame and to first rate movements.

Accordingly, whilst mindfulness leaves the body, fascial elasticity grade by grade recedes as nicely. Typically, regular life throws such a variety of responsibilities at us that we now and again have any time or electricity left for our body. And mindfulness, too, requires strength. We want relaxation to accumulate power and connect with ourselves, to apprehend of noticing with our senses.

Mindfulness is important to find out patterns of physical anxiety and to recognize links with one's mind-set and disposition. These kinds of tensions also can get in the manner of flowing moves. In order to have a look at the types of tension in connection with attitudes and idea strategies, we need eager statement talents and honest self-awareness: Which values are crucial to me? Which desires am I pursuing? Which idea styles do I surely have? And how do those factors change the anxiety in my frame?

This is why Qi Gong trains mindfulness, beginning from easy bodily moves to an increasing number of diffused strategies.

four.Four Why flowing?

We automatically understand flowing movements as lovable and fluid. Such movements may be positioned within the animal usa, in pets and in nicely-educated humans, who keep their our bodies mild and supple. A cat, as an instance, continues its body supple by using the usage of, at the best hand, taking sufficient time to loosen up and doing not anything and, then again, thru executing its actions fluidly. This way that when moves are completed, generally the complete body is concerned. And one movement surely follows the preceding one.

If the movement flows through the whole body, the muscle and fascia tissue learns to coordinate with each different and to paintings together in the fantastic feasible manner. This prevents overexertion of man or woman systems and saves electricity. The movement appears light-footed, supple and flowing. The extra frequently flowing actions are practiced, the more the body gets used to moving with the corresponding performance.

Children additionally carry out movement styles which encompass crawling, walking or hiking very efficiently once they have determined and perfected them – till the primary behavior of anxiety creep in, a number of which copied from parents or constructed up thru strain.

Movements no longer look fluid while too much anxiety receives in the manner and muscle chains/meridians can not take motion. As stated in advance, those muscle chains are interconnected with the useful resource of fascia and stay supple if they're in a position to talk with each other often through anxiety and rest. This is how the mind learns to execute motion styles efficaciously and lightly.

4.5 Why slowly and rapid?

When transferring slowly it's far easier to don't forget and to consciously be privy to a mild, flowing execution of the movements. The greater relaxed the muscle mass are, the better the fascial connections are skilled. Fascia is also capable of take in and launch anxiety, because of this facilitating the interplay of the muscular tissues. By transferring slowly and consciously - as is common in Qi Gong - a feel of connectedness is created during the whole frame. This perceived connectedness with one's very very own nature (one's personal frame) additionally promotes a revel in of connection to and cognizance of nature and the surroundings spherical us.

When appearing rapid moves, the cooperation of the fascial traces worried is critical an amazing way to provide the maximum inexperienced and fast motion feasible. Here, fascia and muscular tissues are harassed for pace. This sports the stability and resistance of the tissues to excessive masses at some point of acceleration and deceleration.

Movement physical sports activities that combine sluggish and rapid actions provide the advantages of each kinds of exercising. But it's far simply as feasible to practice every thing one after the opposite. As for me, I practiced Kung Fu with velocity and Qi Gong at a gradual-motion pace. Some Tai Chi paperwork integrate each modes.

five. Supply of nutrients to

Chapter 3: The Fascia

When it involves fitness, most humans take into account their food plan and nearly every person has probable attempted a diet sooner or later. However, in assessment to the alternative components, workout and respiratory, the food we eat performs a alternatively minor role inside the vitamins of the fascia.

Fasciae aren't furnished without delay with the useful resource of blood vessels, but as an alternative exist as sheaths spherical our cells, muscle corporations, ligaments, organs and bones in a moist surroundings referred to as interstitial fluid, additionally known as lymph. This fluid is in truth located out of doors of the conventional circulatory systems, which includes the blood waft or the drainage of the lymphatic vessels. Although the lymphatic vessels soak up interstitial fluid, they rely upon the assist of the muscle mass as circulatory stimulators.

Fascia works like a sponge that desires to be squeezed occasionally and then launched so that it could replenish with sparkling fluid. Not squeezing the sponge frequently is without a doubt as horrible for the fascia as in no manner letting go.

The interstitial fluid that keeps our fascia supple relies on a sure metabolic turnover to maintain it shifting and regenerating. In one-of-a-type phrases, the musculoskeletal device desires to be moved. If the muscular tissues are going for walks - regardless of the truth that it is genuinely at some stage in a stroll - then the consistent contraction and rest of the numerous muscle mass moreover units the tissue fluid in motion. The muscle tissue push it extra within the path of the pores and pores and skin, in which it may be extra results absorbed via the use of lymph vessels for onward transport. Through the paintings of the cells, substances are in flip excreted into the lymph. This creates a positive skip and renewal of the fluids within the location a few of the cells, wherein the fascia is placed, which gives nutrients for the fascia. In this appreciate, motion is extra crucial than the meals we eat, which wishes to be filtered through the stomach, small gut and massive intestine first.

As continuously, it's miles critical to eat a balanced eating regimen, to put together meals with glowing, natural additives and to pay attention to as a minimum one's very own instinct, although it does no longer in shape into the modern-day tendencies in eating regimen.

Supplements can now and again be beneficial, however they too, like our everyday food, have an prolonged way to go earlier than they achieve the fascia. In addition, the tissue most effective permits itself from the fluid whilst a need is signalled. Bones are an exquisite instance to illustrate this difficulty: No remember how an lousy lot calcium is available within the blood, it is only absorbed whilst the bone cells get preserve of a signal from the musculoskeletal device that the bone goals greater stability. Otherwise, the body does no longer drag round vain weight inside the shape of bone or muscle mass.

The state of affairs is distinct with body fats: it's far accumulated and collected precisely even because it isn't always desired, so that it will prepare for the subsequent 'tough wintry weather' or for the following 'tough healthy dietweight-reduction plan'. The body's ability to shop fat improves further after each a fulfillment food regimen, because the body feels installation: It changed into ultimately very useful to shop the acquired meals as fantastic as viable, for the purpose that a meals deficiency did occur, which has now been triumph over effectively. This is how, amongst different things, the yo-yo effect is created on the identical time as weight loss plan.

It can be assumed that the fluid in the body consists of everything the fascia dreams supplied that one eats a fairly severa weight loss program. Fascia is made of collagen, which consists of protein that the frame can not synthesize itself. This is why the consumption of immoderate outstanding protein is crucial. It is plenty less complex for the body to absorb animal protein than vegetable protein. By ingesting loads of fruit to get nutrients and hint elements, the body additionally receives important fats, fibre and secondary plant materials. These are often lacking whilst taking dietary dietary supplements. Nevertheless, the intake of dietary nutritional supplements can be useful in aggressive sports activities and all through prolonged periods of pressure.

What is essential for fascial elasticity is the fine of the lymphatic fluid, i.E. The fluid that surrounds our cells. Its great, in flip, depends considerably at the nice of our breathing, exercise and nutrients – on this order. Currently, exercise is taken into consideration to be the most critical element for wholesome fascia. Movement feeds the fascia, so to speak. It stimulates the fluids to preserve transferring and eliminates degradation merchandise. Of path, the high-quality of the additives of the fluid in the region between the cells moreover is predicated upon on our everyday healthy dietweight-reduction plan. But the frame's very very own merchandise without a doubt play the more crucial characteristic right proper here, as well as the movement that distributes them as required.

Personally, and I'm absolutely no longer by myself in this, I suspect that the manner we breathe plays a sincere more essential characteristic in nourishing the fascia. Deep, cushty respiratory - this has been seemed for a long term - stimulates the go along with the float of lymph and therefore the drainage of lymphatic fluid. Relaxed breathing will no longer upward thrust up in a highbrow country of tension or pressure. Accordingly, at the identical time as we breathe frivolously the frightened gadget does not motive the frame to supply stress hormones or distinct pressure reactions, which would possibly exchange the chemistry of the body. If the respiratory is calm and deep, the autonomic fearful device is ready to 'rest' and the muscle agencies moreover loosen up extra resultseasily. And comfortable muscle agencies, as I defined in advance than, artwork collectively greater harmoniously. Movements become smoother and additional green. Fewer blockages boom. And all this truely thru breathing in a calm, comfortable manner.

It is consequently now not surprising that the breath plays this type of important role in ancient fitness practices which include yoga, meditation and Qi Gong.

On Qi Gong

1. What is Qi Gong?

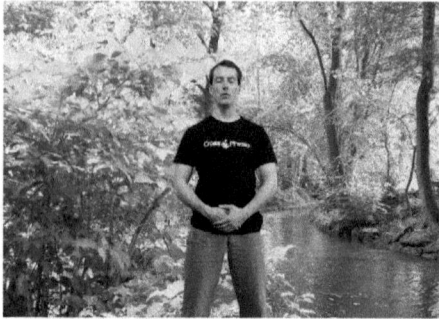

Qi Gong is a relaxing, aware exercising shape from China that still works at the anxious gadget thru gradual, rhythmic motion and law of the breath. By manner of the autonomic anxious device, the muscle tissues return to a cushty u.S.A.. The moderate moves as a result make a contribution to the regeneration of the fascia.

Qi Gong does now not stretch individual muscle mass, but gently encourages muscle and fascia chains to artwork together, making moves every greater efficient and clean. Joints are moved three-dimensionally, in contrast to what is frequently done within the gymnasium on machines. Qi Gong physical video video games additionally incorporate the breath and mindfulness.

Because its effect on everyday fitness is so profound, Qi Gong is one of the 5 pillars of Traditional Chinese Medicine.

Qi Gong bodily sports activities set off in which there can be too little tension and release wherein there can be too much anxiety. The sports activities are extensively speaking finished at the same time as reputation, on occasion whilst sitting or mendacity down. They usually have a pleasant effect at the alignment of the backbone. It is then feasible to preserve an upright posture with no trouble and for an prolonged time period. An upright posture goes hand in hand with natural, comfortable and full respiratory. However, our posture is often affected by severa vain tension, which then also has a terrible impact on our respiratory sample.

Even emotional tensions can be released at the same time as the focal point is directed faraway from beyond memories or modern suffering and alternatively movements towards independent or splendid components of lifestyles through mindfulness. This is why Qi

Gong is likewise used for burnout prevention, for instance.

Practicing Qi Gong can consequently release physical, similarly to highbrow tension. Physical and mental tension are frequently related besides.

Breathing is cautiously linked to our posture: the external, bodily posture of the spine in addition to our inner, highbrow posture. It is less tough to respire glaringly when the outer posture is comfortable and upright and the anxiety within the muscle groups is capable of adapt freely to the situation, i.E. Can release. If the breath flows obviously and freely, the thoughts moreover turns into smooth and calm. This creates a aware spirit that perceives and directs the frame, but does not restrain it. This can then purpose in addition - deep internal - relaxation.

Confucius is mentioned to have stated:

"First placed yourself so as, then your circle of relatives, and then society."

From this aspect of view, Qi Gong permits the practitioner in putting themselves so as and to then enforce this order externally (family and society). Internal order starts with the calming of the breath and the rest of the body. Appropriate contemplation of the times of lifestyles (a philosophy) permits the frame to loosen up. Qi Gong is most often associated with philosophies in conjunction with Taoism or Buddhism. These philosophies can function a device for our thoughts to higher integrate the sports into our every day lifestyles, to understand them as a herbal a part of ourselves and to use them as a useful aid. Equally beneficial, but, are reflections and insights from super psychology and comparable fields.

A clean, nicely-knowledgeable thoughts is crucial as a way to live lifestyles consciously. It makes it less difficult to differentiate among what is critical and what's superfluous. What do I really need to be content?

Usually it takes numerous years to transport from the physical degree of working in the direction of the sports to a in reality deep, profound relaxation of frame and mind. Then the mind becomes clear like a peaceful lake and fact may be perceived anew, just like children definitely do. However, this can moreover be professional inside the very first consultation. Being able to lighten up deeply is in itself not some thing special.

1.1 The four degrees of internal workout

The schooling of Qi Gong can be more or a good deal less divided into 4 areas.

These are:

-

 body

-

 breath

-

 psyche / coronary coronary heart / emotion

-

 mind

The following description may additionally moreover moreover seem great within the beginning. But with growing practice it will make feel to you:

At first I recognition greater at the body, with questions like: "What is the right stance? Why are my thighs straining lots? Why can't I permit pass of the tension in my neck?"

Then I increasingly more direct my focus to the breath: "Can't I exhale and inhale extra slowly? Why do I keep dropping recognition on my breath? Again, I've been preserving my breath in vicinity of letting it glide."

After training for a while, emotions begin to arise. The frame is relatively cushty, the breath flows with the movement. Emotions are attacking our recognition on doing the smooth physical video games. However, every sorts of feelings - terrible in addition to great - are virtually distractions, 'twitches of the nerves' which may be discharged in the tranquility of the workout.

Eventually, the feelings have settled down and the mind is busy with itself. Trains of mind study each other: "Oh, my emotions are without a doubt calm, I can revel in the workout. How splendidly diligent I am. I genuinely have determined my manner, I, I, I ..."

This maintains till there's actually simply reputation. Nothing greater. Meaning, the whole lot else is there too, but now not a lot in the focus. At that 2nd, our belief can enter into our recognition in a renewed way. The ego stands with the aid of the usage of the usage of and is used increasingly more for the obligations which may be in reality important and does no longer continuously intervene within the whole factor.

In order no longer to wander away in spiritual-mental dreams as one progresses, a personal courting with an skilled trainer is commonly very important.

2. Qi Gong to train the fascia

When searching at Qi Gong carrying activities in terms of fascial schooling, it speedy will become clear that those ancient bodily games contain many critical components of what makes an first rate fascial exercise. Without modern-day medical expertise, doctors in earlier times relied on the art work of remark. A supple, bendy and robust body remains considered the right in Asia. This first-class is also based totally on what can be determined in nature. As a surrender result, many sporting sports in Qi Gong to within the in the meantime imitate animal features, on the facet of the agility of a snake, the stableness of a crane, or the monkey's ease of jumping.

Using the language of Traditional Chinese Medicine, Qi Gong improves the go with the flow of energies via the frame. In modern-day-day phrases, Qi Gong mainly mobilizes the primary fascial strands (muscle chains) and lets in to extend healthful, bendy fascia. Such healthy fascia is wet and have to be stored hydrated and lubricated thru movement. Failure to carry out that could result in adhesions and tears within the fascial shape.

The go along with the waft of fluids among the muscle fibres and connective tissue membranes should consequently no longer be blocked, specifically along the fundamental, crucial muscle chains (meridians). Otherwise, there may be reduced functionality, i.E. Overall general performance loss, or perhaps ache. Qi Gong has constantly been geared inside the route of these fascial characteristic chains, besides that human beings in historic China did now not understand them and therefore referred to as them otherwise, i.E. Meridians. In his ebook 'Anatomy Trains', Tom Myers describes the fascial muscle chains in element. He carefully refers to the similarity to the Chinese meridians as 'coincidental'. With this anatomical view of the Asian meridians as a vantage point, the bodily sports grow to be an lousy lot less hard to get entry to and apprehend. Many things that before the whole thing seem uncertain inside the traditional language of Qi Gong will then unexpectedly end up smooth to understand, and allow for a sincere deeper facts.

In a more current ebook thru Robert Schleip with the become aware of 'Fascia in Sport and Everyday Life', visitor writer Chia writes that he assumes that the oh-so-mysterious Qi may moreover glide via the fascial tissue – especially if Qi is referred to as flowing life energy. A person's Qi may want to hence be synonymous with the current-day u.S.A. Of america of their fascial tissue. If the fascia is supple and unfastened, the Qi, i.E. The lifestyles power, is able to waft well – life energy in the revel in of flowing strain transmission through the meridians/muscle chains and the change of the fluids within the connective tissue. A blockage of Qi ought to because of this be equal to sticky fascia. And each may be launched via the moderate movements of Qi Gong, acupressure or rubdown.

Here, Qi Gong affects the fascia on one in each of a kind stages: at the only hand, in a only mechanical way via the slight, three-dimensional moves, but instead, moreover through the nervous machine. The slow movements calm the worried system, the breath deepens and the muscle tone decreases.

In this second the fascia can get higher from assets of pressure. In different phrases, Qi Gong stimulates regeneration thru inducing a comfortable nation of the annoying tool.

In ancient China they'll have spoken of releasing 'Qi blockages', today we are able to use the term 'fascial adhesions'. So Qi Gong may also be referred to as 'Fascia Gong': working on the fascia.

With this in mind, it is straightforward to apprehend Qi Gong training as a very modern-day fascia training. It promotes tenderness, suppleness, attention and mindfulness, calms the worried device and stimulates the metabolism.

These well-designed physical sports are capable of efficaciously assisting many critical systems in our body.

three. Studies on Qi Gong

More and greater research attest to the benefits of Qi Gong. It is consequently now not sudden that Qi Gong is also increasingly more finding its manner into scientific centres within the west to supplement the sort of restoration tactics on provide there.

A look at published in 2010 summarized all formerly published English-language studies and listed the results of Qi Gong and its relative Tai Chi. It suggests that every Asian exercising applications have examined pleasant effects in the following areas:

•mental symptoms and signs and symptoms

•prevention of falls

•cardiopulmonary tool

•nice of lifestyles

•functioning of the musculoskeletal gadget

•self-efficacy/resilience

•immune tool

•bone density

All the ones structures are essential for the body's power deliver or for energy distribution within the frame.

Another examine investigated the consequences of Qi Gong on continual pain and got here to the belief that the wearing activities have a pain-relieving impact and also have excellent consequences on associated signs and symptoms and symptoms consisting of sleep top notch, urge for food, capacity to pay attention, and so forth.

A vital have a have a have a look at examined the results of preceding studies on Qi Gong with respect to Fibromyalgia. It emphasizes the effectiveness of Qi Gong, however states that the effectiveness correlates with the intensity of exercising and the strength of mind of the participants, which might be frequently no longer documented as it want to be. The extra time and depth of the exercise will increase, the more truly the fulfillment of the sports sports suggests.

It can therefore be stated that, beyond the best subjective feeling of the physical sports being high-quality and fun, Qi Gong has been set up to have many normal health benefits, to reduce pain and to promote regeneration. By freeing fascial adhesions, selling an prolonged and lively existence, Qi Gong therefore contributes to retaining our bodies supple, flexible and limber.

Links to the research may be determined at the give up of the ebook within the bibliography and link listing.

four. Traditional Chinese Medicine in evaluation with Western biopsychosocial remedy.

TCM is an empirical scientific device that has superior over hundreds of years. In assessment, biopsychosocial treatment stays quite more youthful. It emerged in the middle of the ultimate century as a counter-motion to the increasingly more technical surgical remedy. Its holistic techniques resemble TCM's aspect of view, however they will be primarily based on the medical worldview of Western remedy, on the equal time because the concepts of TCM have been before everything based totally on non secular-philosophical international views.

Both scientific schools study people now not simplest bodily from pinnacle to backside, but moreover maintain in mind their emotional u . S ., lifestyle behavior, and social relationships. For professional practitioners of every models, a whole lot of that is contemplated within the affected man or woman's physical scenario.

A demystified version of TCM is currently taught on the Heidelberg School of Prof. Greten. This college acknowledges the big have an effect on the worrying tool has at the affected individual and uses the strategies of TCM to have the capacity to persuade and control it.

Fascia researchers are also interested in TCM. They have placed that within the region close to the needling, acupuncture has an impact at the fascial tissues. Furthermore, many TCM rubdown techniques are similar to Western massage strategies centered on the fascia and connective tissue. Research shows that after the cells in the fascial connective tissue are stimulated, they launch neurotransmitters that make contributions to the frame's relaxation. Emotional stress, which formerly might also have manifested as anxiety within the connective tissue, is launched in this way.

An professional TCM therapist will acquire a holistic picture of the apprehensive device and pick out applicable triggering elements. In this manner, ache can be handled in a symptom-oriented manner and reasons which is probably placed out of doors the frame may be diagnosed. Qi Gong carrying sports can be advocated and life-style changes is probably referred to as a way to beautify the affected individual's popular circumstance and cause them to extra resilient.

This technique is just like that of a therapist knowledgeable in biopsychosocial treatment. In my opinion, biopsychosocial medicine may be understood as a bridge to TCM. Many studies consequences from biopsychosocial treatment can be used to higher understand TCM, specifically outcomes from fascia research and psychoneuroimmunology. If techniques and techniques from TCM can be understood in this manner, it makes it less complicated to recognize and integrate it into technological know-how-primarily based virtually treatment.

So fascia no longer best connects character organs and physical abilities to form a coherent machine – it moreover bridges the distance between jap, traditional medication (TCM) and western, era-primarily based medicine.

The reality that the frame does now not artwork independently from its imperative unit, our mind, changed into already known in ancient China. Today, the effects of emotional pressure on fascial tissue can be defined with the assist of the concerned device and its neurotransmitters. Back then, one should sincerely see the outcomes: Stress results in anxiety and modifications inside the tissue, relying on how the individual in question professional the stress. This gave upward push to an in depth philosophy of existence whose purpose to in recent times is to make humans independent and resilient within the face of outside affects. These mental elements of Taoist-Buddhist philosophy are increasingly more finding their way into the contemporary restoration environment. Techniques for developing mindfulness have come to be increasingly well-known and feature the capability to have an effect on all regions of life.

Practical issue: The 5 most

Chapter 4: Effective Qi Gong Bodily Activities For The Fascia

1. Before you exercising

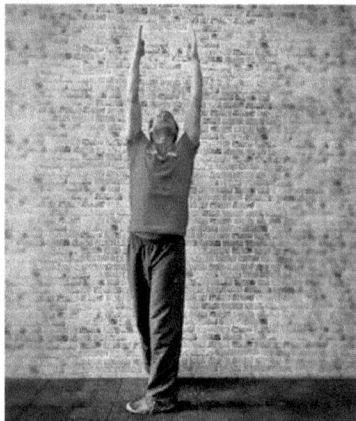

1.1 When to exercise?

Any time of day is fine. Early mornings or evenings are suitable. Times at which matters calm down. It is vital to exercise regularly, as that is the only manner to deepen the exercise.

1.2 When not to exercise?

If you enjoy ill, it's far better to take a destroy from workout. After eating, you need to wait as a minimum half of of-hour in advance than workout.

1.Three What to put on?

Comfortable, warm clothing is important. A converting ritual also can assist to set the temper for the exercise.

1.Four Where to exercising?

Ideally out of doors, or in a quiet room. If important, you need to permit others understand that you do no longer need to be disturbed.

1.5 Do I must warm up?

Warming up is crucial for the frame and it prepares the muscle tissue and joints for the paintings earlier. If feasible, half of the education time need to be used to heat up. This will make the following sports smoother and plenty much less complex to consolidate. For the bodily sports provided proper proper right here, a quick stroll or taking some flights of stairs up or down will do. If that isn't feasible, you can stroll immediate for a few minutes or pat your body collectively along with your hands.

To warmness up, you could use what I name Paleo sporting events. More data can be observed on my internet website.

1.6 What in case you abruptly ought to prevent?

That' s no longer a hassle. Simply pause the workout and retain later. In famous, but, it's miles higher now not to be interrupted in the course of the exercising. So it's far top notch to position your cell cellphone and different gadgets on silent.

1.7 Breathing correctly

During the workout of Qi Gong, you have to not try and pressure a selected respiratory. Just allow the breath glide freely internal and out. Even although there are respiration instructions for some bodily video games, the ones must now not be accompanied compulsively. The component, ultimately, is to step by step lighten up via the exercise, simply so the breath glaringly becomes calm and deep. Frantically searching out to deepen and prolong it, most effective reasons new tensions. That's why I advise to pay hobby at the flow of movement in the beginning and becoming slower and calmer in the approach.

1.8 How lots to practice?

If feasible: 5 to ten minutes every day, then the movement sequences will consolidate. Relaxation may even slowly deepen, grow to be less difficult and additional surely possible. Don't be too strict with yourself. Daily can also translate into practicing five out of seven days in keeping with week. Or you could determine to exercise 2 instances in step with week - if that appears greater practical - and then be constant with it.

If you workout each day, you ought to see the number one successes after approximately 3 weeks, in the texture that you're feeling more cushty and are capable to call in this experience in demanding situations.

1.Nine Is the collection of the sporting events crucial?

The bodily games listed underneath can be practiced in any order, or you can do truely simply one among them. The only important aspect is which you discover a regular workout everyday, preferably a few minutes each day.

2. My 5 most effective Qi Gong carrying sports for the fascia

2.1 The Flying Dragon – for a sturdy and flexible backbone

The most herbal and free shape of exercise for the fascia is dancing with abandon, as it has been practiced thinking about that ancient times, as an instance, round a campfire. Here, the frame is moved rhythmically and in all instructions. Modern ballroom dance, which includes retaining the spine stiff, isn't always what is supposed proper proper right here. The concept is for our spine to turn out to be a vertebral snake over again. The calm yet powerful exercising The Flying Dragon is

 very suitable for this cause.

To practice The Flying Dragon, you neither want track nor precise feeling for rhythm. The workout has a cushty, invigorating effect on the capability and power of the backbone. It is pretty strenuous at the begin, however you can quickly be rewarded with the sensation of being able to bypass extra with out issue.

Tutorial: The Flying Dragon

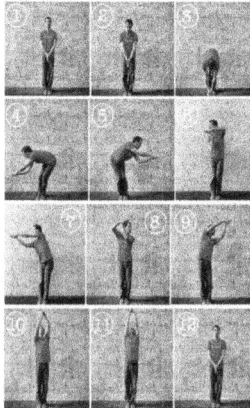

1. Stand at the aspect of your toes near together (see Figure 1). If that is too tough, place your feet shoulder-width apart.

2. Bring your arms together and hold them in competition to every exclusive any more.

3. Lower your top frame till your fingertips contact the floor. If you can't bend down that low, pause in brief at the factor in that you feel you cannot skip any in addition. In this in advance fold feature, in brief try and relax your

shoulders, neck, and lower again. The knees ought to though stay absolutely prolonged. However, if there's too much tension inside the knees on this selection, you could bend them slightly. Inhale and exhale deeply some instances, with arms and head setting down closer to the floor. (Figure 2 and 3)

four. Now start the flight of the dragon. Imagine that your folded arms are the dragon's head. Point the dragon head, which changed into pointing downward the complete time, to the left and fly your fingertips as a long way to the left as your backbone allows. The knees in the mean time are bent. Let the dragon's head take off as low as viable. This technique that it will fly near the ground inside the starting. When the mobility of the spine and shoulders is maxed out and it cannot cross any further to the side, the dragon head, i.E. The fingertips, turns spherical. It then flies lower back a hint better and to the alternative aspect — continually extra or a bargain much less parallel to the floor. At the prevent of the movement, the dragon's head turns spherical and flies slowly a bit higher and better, like a chook close to a mountain slope which makes use of the upwind drafts to upward push up. Repeat this 3 or four times. Ideally, if you started out out out together with your fingertips on the ground, you could have flown like this as quickly as to knee height, then to hip top, then chest height, and eventually to face peak. Once proper right here, turn your fingertips inside the course of the ceiling and fly collectively collectively along with your fingers proper away up, stretching your complete frame. Again, stay on this function for some breaths. (Figure 4 to eleven)

5. Once your fingertips have reached the uppermost position and you have in quick sensed the overall extension of your frame, lower the fingertips/head of the dragon from the very top right away and slowly down inside the front of your body till you're yet again on the region to begin inside the lowest feature you could acquire. Extend your legs again right right here and in quick try and lighten up your drooping palms and head. (Figure 12, then 1 to 3)

6. Then bend your knees slightly and repeat the flying dragon series three to 10 times in a row. Perform the actions as slowly and mindfully as feasible. Do now not stress yourself to respire flippantly. Breathe as is herbal for you. (Figure 4 and following)

2.2 The Bear – for robust shoulders and belly

Before we've got a have a look at to walk on legs as infants, we very well prepare our muscular tissues to reap this by using the use of crawling substantially on all fours. This moreover strengthens, stabilizes and mobilizes the spine. This primal shape of exercise is likewise finding more and more reputation inside the health international. If your hands have not been used to assist your self at the floor for a long time, The Bear may be difficult within the beginning. So take some time. Do short exercising classes best and get better sufficiently earlier than doing some other series of sporting sports.

Tutorial: The Bear

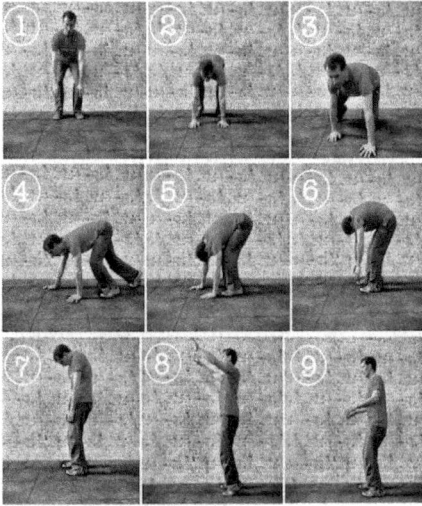

1. Stand along with your toes shoulder-width apart, knees barely bent. Lower your higher frame till your palms are touching the ground and you may lean on your hands. You can bend your knees as you try this. (Figure 1 and multiple)

2. Now first circulate a ways from your feet together with your hands. When you have reached a snug distance, skip forwards, backwards or sideways on all fours. Try different things. Each time you convey one hand off the floor, make sure to loosen up the shoulder of that arm in advance than shifting

your weight decrease lower back onto it. Walk slowly and mindfully. Imagine you're a bear roaming a flowery clearing, curiously noticing precise shapes, shades, and smells. (Figure three and 4)

three. Do now not do that workout for too prolonged, especially inside the beginning, in order now not to overload your shoulders. Instead, take a quick damage after a quick schooling consultation or practice a miles less tough exercise after which come lower decrease back to this exercise. With developing exercising you could find that you could teach for longer at a stretch and additionally expand the distance amongst feet and palms increasingly, due to the fact the power within the better body and torso increases.

To end the workout, skip your palms and ft once more collectively. Then shift your weight truly onto your toes so you can increase your hands. Slowly roll the backbone upward, straightening vertebra through vertebra. (Figure 6 and 7)

Then, whilst you're reputation upright over again, shift your weight beforehand onto the balls of your toes and raise your heels off the ground. Raise your fingers barely above shoulder pinnacle. Bend the fingers like claws. Then decrease your palms all over again and relax. (Figure eight and nine)

2.Three The Eagle – balance schooling and rest for shoulders and breath

This exercising is inspired by using the majestic grace of an eagle status excessive up on a ledge, starting its wings to cool its body. As it does so, it stands on one leg and gazes a ways into the gap.

One the great hand, this exercise is set enhancing stability on one leg, and on the opportunity approximately a laugh the shoulders and chest. The more relaxed the shoulders and chest are, the a great deal much less complicated we breathe. Imagine if the lungs had been in a rigid cage, as they're at the equal time as the vertebrae and ribs are stiff and tight. Breathing would be very difficult. But if the ribs, vertebrae and mild tissue at some stage in the rib cage can bypass freely, it is hundreds much less complex for the lungs to make entire use in their respiration quantity.

During this workout, make certain to commonly maintain your legs barely bent. Depending on how proper your stability is, you could pick different versions of the workout. In the beginning it's far less complex with each legs at the ground. Later, bring one leg and if that works well, you can even close to your eyes in some unspecified time in the future of the exercising.

Tutorial: The Eagle

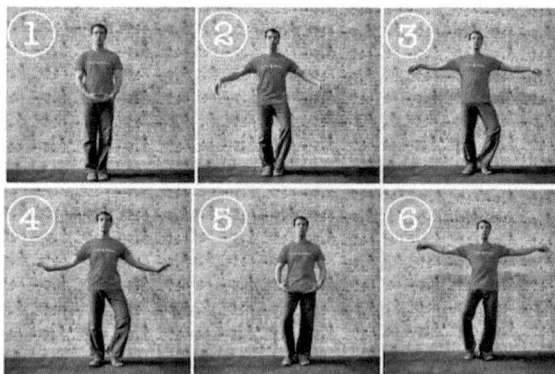

1. Stand together with your legs together and bring your arms within the front of your

decrease abdomen. One hand lies on pinnacle of the alternative. It makes no distinction to your fascia whether or not your left hand is on pinnacle of your right or the opportunity manner round. In some traditional faculties, symbolic meanings are associated with the palms, inclusive of male and lady. This can be massive for extremely advanced practitioners. To start with, just do it within the way that feels maximum snug to you, or change the hands in case you enjoy like it. (Figure 1)

2. Now separate your hands and flow into your fingers outwards so they spread out like fowl's wings. The arms have to barely hold down from the wrists, as even though the palms were lifted via threads associated with the wrists. As you do that, shift your weight to as a minimum one leg. Lift the opportunity leg barely truly so handiest the ball of the foot lightly touches the ground, with out truely setting any weight on it. The leg on which the body weight now rests is called the 'full leg'. The distinct is the 'empty leg'. If you revel in confident about your balance, you can in brief deliver the empty leg clearly off the ground. When you decrease the

leg decrease again to the ground, make sure you do it as lightly and slowly as possible. (Figure 2 and 3)

3. When your fingers attain about shoulder pinnacle even as elevating your fingers, reverse the movement. Make notable, mainly at this second, that your shoulders are cushty and your elbows are barely bent. When the palms then start the downward motion, component the fingertips upward as though the arms actually need to push the air out from under them. Continue to lower them and place the hands lower lower back on pinnacle of every unique at the level of your lower belly. (Figure 4 and 1)

4. In this manner, enhance and reduce your arms like eagle wings 3 instances on the same time as balancing at the identical leg.

5. Switch to the opposite leg best after the 3rd time and then repeat the gathering all over again: growth and reduce your palms three instances, then shift your weight to the empty leg. Make sure to continuously preserve the knee of the popularity leg barely bent. Repeat this exercising approximately 9 to 30 instances

– in exclusive phrases, increase and decrease your arms nine to 30 instances. Always drift slowly and breathe as is snug for you. (Figure five and 6 display the proper leg because the 'empty leg')

2.Four Standing Still – deep relaxation and breathing

Does status however train the fascia? While this could sound contradictory in advance than the whole thing, it is very powerful training for the fascia – in a completely unique way than the movement bodily sports. By status nevertheless without any actual cause, tensions are released and our respiratory calms down. This deep, internal relaxation is communicated through the involved tool to all the fibres of our frame: it is now time to relaxation and regenerate. Relaxation is an crucial element of training. Just like muscular tissues grow within the resting intervals as quickly as you have got stimulated through way of a exercising, fascia will begin to make bigger areas which can be used loads and will decrease the anxiety of their contractile factors. Consequently, this shape of deep, internal rest is also part of an effective fascial exercise. As our frightened tool switches from regular fight or flight mode to relaxation and digest mode, those indicators boosting our regenerative techniques are taken up everywhere in the body.

This aware shift from activity to regeneration isn't always smooth to study, but has many benefits for one's very very personal fitness and for a top notch autonomy and independence concerning one's private self care, surely so I would really like to endorse this exercising to everyone. There is a motive why it's far been practiced for hundreds of years and may be decided in almost all varieties of Qi Gong and additionally other martial arts.

For the workout, stand though, like a tree. Only the breath lightly movements your top body. You will possibly moreover observe which you aren't repute despite the fact that and motionless like a statue the least bit, however lightly swaying round your body's centre of gravity, like a tree shifting with the wind.

Chapter 5: Tutorial: Standing Still

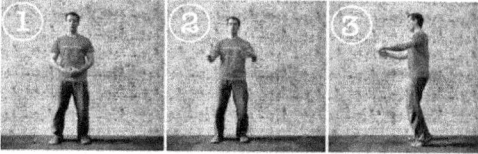

1. Stand collectively with your toes shoulder-width apart and your knees barely bent constantly. Tilt your pelvis so that your decrease lower returned is flat, i.E. Your lower lower back isn't always arched.

2. Straighten your better frame as although a thread end up pulling you up at the crown of your head. Open your mouth big a few times to loosen your jaw. Then region your lips together ever so lightly.

3. Variation A:

Place your palms in your decrease belly with one hand on pinnacle of the alternative. Shoulders and elbows are genuinely comfortable. (Figure 1)

3. Variation B:

Raise your palms within the the front of your torso. The fingers aspect type of in the route of the sternum or belly. Thumbs element upward, as even though your fingers have been held in role with the useful resource of using a thread on your thumbs. While doing this, hold your wrists, elbows and shoulders as snug as possible. (Figure 2)

three. Variation C:

Arms like in Variation B. In addition, shift your weight all of the manner ahead onto the balls of your feet simply so your heels are lifted. This workout additionally trains balance and power inside the calf muscle tissue. Hold this stance as long as you can. However, do not overdo it. When your muscle organizations get tired, rest. (Figure 3)

4. Close your eyes if you like. Feel in which your weight creates tension to your frame. In Variation A and B, shift your body weight so you enjoy it to your foot right above the metatarsus, or similarly in the the front. You must no longer experience the primary weight for your heels.

5. You can now truely stay in the respective function and feature a look at yourself. Set yourself a timer and stay in one of the reputation poses above for five-10 mins.

five.1. While you live however in one position, repeat the subsequent respiratory workout 10 times in a row:

Exhale through barely closed lips on 'FFFFFF-T'. The prolonged 'FFFFF' sound should set off your belly, with the intention to then assist to push the air from your lungs as you exhale. The quick 'T' at the end must specifically activate the diaphragm all over again. After the 'FFFFFF-T', leave your mouth open in order that the air can go together with the go with the flow in on its very very personal in some unspecified time within the destiny of the following herbal reflex to inhale. When doing this, do no longer pressure the air into your lungs. Let your frame do its artwork. You will observe that after exhaling, your lungs inhale occasionally more shallow and from time to time more deeply. When you're finished with this breathing exercising, preserve to stand even though and breathe glaringly.

2.Five Metal Exercise – stretching the backbone in a spiral shape

This workout originates from the 5 elements exercise in Qi Gong. The tension that is held in short on the give up, from the end of the toes to the fingertips stretched a protracted way upwards, symbolizes the detail metal. Metal represents regeneration and powerful breathing. The chest is stretched and opened, the shoulders are lifted all of the way up. The stretch extends via the hips to the suggestions of the feet. Tension and relaxation trade. The mild rotation to the side, with the recognition leg unmoving, creates a moderate diagonal pull in the frame, which consequently stimulates the helix-ordinary fascial connections.

Tutorial: Metal Exercise

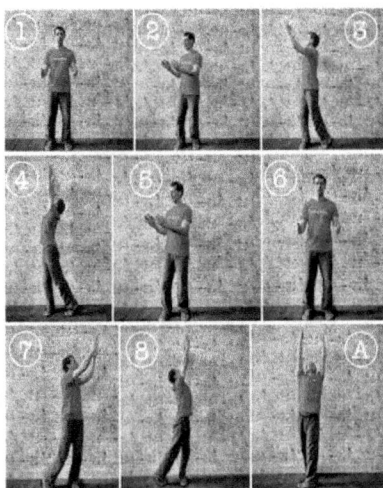

1. Stand on the facet of your ft shoulder-width aside. Raise your palms in front of your torso at the facet of your palms managing every distinctive. Your fingers want to regardless of the fact that be snug.

(Figure 1)

2. Now flip your better body to the facet, for example to the proper. The proper leg remains in area as it's miles. Only the leg this is now inside the lower back rotates with your torso, the heel lifting and simplest the hints of the toes keeping contact with the ground. (Figure 2 and three)

3. Raise your palms up in the the front of you as some distance as you could, collectively together with your hands going thru every unique. Now together with your palms handling every distinct, tighten them barely as if you have been keeping a heavy stone amongst them. The tension need to be felt at some point of your hand all the way for your fingertips. When you reach the pinnacle, pause for a few breaths and enjoy the anxiety stretching out of your lower back feet thru the arc of your body to your fingertips. (Figure four)

four. Relax your palms and shoulders and slowly flow once more to the start feature, arms although going through each other. (Figure 5 and 6)

five. Then flip your torso to the left. This time, the left leg remains as it turned into inside the beginning function. While rotating to the left, now the proper leg rotates and is lifting barely until exceptional the toes or the ball of the foot is in touch with the floor. Raise, straighten and tighten the fingers once more as in step three.

(Figure 7 and eight; Figure A shows the very last role from the aspect)

6. Practice the gathering of moves as slowly as you could. Consciously loosen up every time you return to the start feature. Repeat every factor five to 10 times.

three. Learning the artwork of doing no longer something – rest within the animal usa

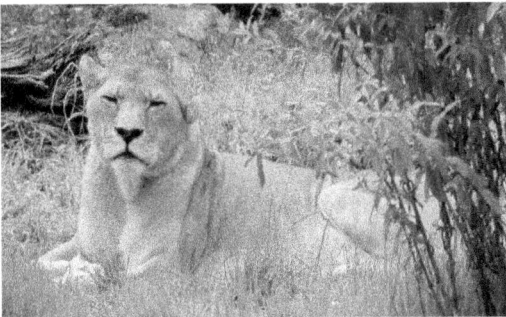

When animals flow into, we respect their suppleness and energy. We test the animal in its movement and can use it to growth bodily activities for our very private our our our bodies. However, we often overlook how an lousy lot time animals spend in easy terms doing not anything and searching after their frame. How many hours does a tiger spend lying within the color of a tree? How many hours do monkeys sit or lie inside the grass or in tree branches? How lots time do they spend in cushty assertion?

Especially nowadays - while the entirety is geared in the direction of basic performance and there can be an app for every hobby to enhance our performance - it's far critical to don't forget that we want everyday instances of rest. Moments wherein we will honestly have a observe without having to pursue a motive. Perhaps we ought to also be capable of go through moments of boredom.

Most of what we do appears to be incredible a way to an give up. An stop that has imposed itself ultimately, that springs from a combination of upbringing and social strain.

Would it is justifiable to spend a 2d with none useful interest? Or even an entire day, an entire week? Well, what is it like inside the animal united states?

The tiger will visit the watering hollow while it feels thirsty. If its thirst is quenched, it will lie down over again in its spot or roam its territory. Once it has had eaten its fill, it rests sufficiently. Hunger pushes it to are searching for for at the right time. It does no longer hunt for the cause of resting afterwards, nor does it relaxation on the way to be able to successfully hunt later. It follows the requirements of the instant and is for this reason gift with all its senses.

Are we ever in this sort of country of natural presence? Already as children, we shift our attention increasingly to requirements and mind as we become older. This is because of the complexities of social existence and its have an effect on on our mind hobby. Our thoughts produces snap shots of our future and aligns our movements therefore. There isn't something wrong with this: It allows us to devise and act thoughtfully and is a fantastic human achievement. However, the task is not to lose the capability to revel in and revel in moments with our senses. As adults, this inherently natural functionality, which each toddler is born with, frequently needs to be actively relearned.

So permit's once in a while turn inwards, close to our eyes and experience what we need in that second. With Qi Gong we skip lightly within the 2d, with out externally visible results. For a 2d we become easy and susceptible, just so the body is capable of regenerate, loose from motive and obligation.

As a character, am I actually at liberty to try this?

I could say: As someone, I want to take this liberty! Otherwise I act like a device, totally worried with best my duties. This is particularly tempting inside the age of optimization.

So Qi Gong is a form of 'doing not anything' that is (partly) mounted via society. Granted, we are analyzing more and more approximately the health advantages of Qi Gong, which contributes in addition to social popularity and enables to encourage us to exercise till it has grow to be a everyday a part of our lives that we perform as a recollect variety of direction just like brushing our tooth within the morning.

Those who discover as 'doers' find out it specially hard to relate to Qi Gong. From the outside, no longer a bargain truely takes location at the equal time as doing Qi Gong: A man or woman is reputation within the coloration of a tree, eyes closed. They float one arm in slow motion, moving their weight from one leg to the alternative. What has took place after 10 mins? Nothing. What stays after the workout? Nothing. Possibly a pleasant 'now not something'. So what became the motive of the exercise? The 'now not something'?

Yes, no longer some thing, without a doubt, within the enjoy of our person 'point 0'. Just being there. No anxiety. No combat. No flight. No cause. Breathing. Observing – if you want to name that cause. In this enjoy, the 'nothingness' only applies to our chattering thoughts, which nearly continuously assets us with requirements, stressful motives that soak up all our attention and leave no room for the processing of present moments and sensory impressions.

Everything else keeps at the equal time as we're doing no longer something: we breathe, we stand, our senses are aware and our heart is pumping. Shifting our mindfulness to the ones 'inanimate' strategies can energize us plenty. With energy this is otherwise made available to and absorbed by means of idea processes.

This nothingness may also be known as our natural 'being', the deliver of our being. All thoughts come from this 'nothingness', from being. It is the breeding ground and additionally the deliver of electricity for all our moves and thoughts.

Chapter 6: Hold In A Positive Course

You can remember the connection of fascia in the equal way as a station, a railroad tune, a turntable, and so forth.

The running muscle businesses and tendons are like railroad tracks, and the attachments of muscle tendons are like stations and switches.

Like a real educate, the fascial connection have to each run immediately or alternate route in small increments in order for the fascial connection to transmit anxiety.

The fascial connection want to moreover move straight away or have a slight curve just so the train can not turn ninety ° at proper angles at the equal time as the usage of.

Also, it isn't always possible to alternate to other fascias with brilliant muscle depths as in the actual teach. As a favored rule, unexpected turns and depth adjustments deviate from the principle.

When this takes area, the transmission of anxiety due to the fascia will no longer feature.

For example, the pectoralis minor and coracobrachialis are related by means of manner of the use of fascia.

It is fascially linked, but while the arm is down, the 2 muscle organizations are going via in without a doubt considered certainly one of a kind pointers, so it does no longer feature as an fascial connection in any respect.

However, whilst you increase your hand like a badminton harm, the pectoralis minor and coracobrachialis muscles are linked in a immediately line, so the fascial connection works from the ribs to the fingers.

When you take a posture to be able to boom your shoulders and hangs, you may increase your alternatives whether or no longer it is because of the above muscle troubles or thing due to muscle connection (other muscle groups on the anatomy train).

In the example of the pectoralis minor and coracobrachialis, those muscle mass are the Connection of fascia inside the deep layers of the body within the fascial connection.

It is going from the thumb via the radius and biceps to the pectoralis minor.

In the above posture, it additionally connects to the superficial anterior fascia and additionally to the rectus abdominis muscle.

From this, within the case of the pectoralis minor and coracobrachialis muscle tissues, it's far viable that the motion is affected from the better limbs via the shoulders to the abdomen to the pelvis.

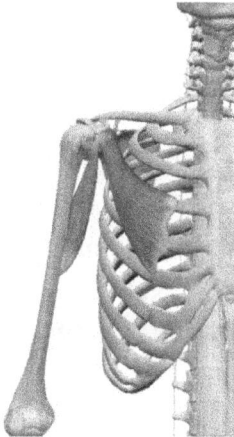

There are exceptions to the course of the fascial connection, and the fibula muscle organizations bend at proper angles from the outer ankle via the bone, however in this example they act like pulleys and art work in line with the regulation.

This is a the front view of the pectoralis minor and coracobrachialis muscle tissue at the proper issue.

When the arm is dwindled, there's a steep mindset some of the muscular tissues and it does not feature as an fascial connection, however at the same time as the shoulder joint is raised, the muscle companies be a part of and characteristic as an anatomy train.

Muscle intensity is also essential.

For instance, whilst the trunk and neck are extended backwards, the rectus abdominis muscle and the infrahyoid muscle in the throat are stretched, so it seems that there is a muscle connection, but in fact it's far one among a kind.

The rectus abdominis muscle is attached to the sternalis muscle and sternocleidomastoid muscle as a superficial anterior fascia, and the infrahyoid muscle is attached to the intrathoracic fascia deep inside the sternum.

The purpose for this is that the layers in which the muscle groups run are specific.

This is a the the front view of the rectus abdominis muscle, sternalis muscle, and sternocleidomastoid muscle at the proper trouble.

It seems that the rectus abdominis muscle $\Rightarrow$ sternum muscle is mounted from the pubis to the infrahyoid muscle that extends at once up.

But, in truth from the muscle layer difference it'll bring about the sternocleidomastoid muscle that is at the outdoor.

The infrahyoid muscle, however, connects to the fascia within the returned of the sternum.

Also, according to the anatomy teach regulation, the anatomy train may not be shaped in spite of the fact that the muscular tissues run and attach together.

For instance, the adductor longus and biceps femoris brachycephaly meet the requirements of the anatomy teach. But in fact, for Ouchi adductor muscle is present between the 2 of muscle, no state of affairs is glad.

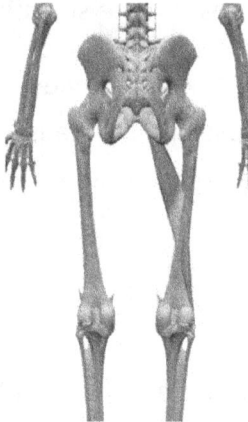

This is an image of the adductor longus muscle and the brachycephaly of the biceps femoris seen from the returned.

 With the femur in among, it seems like it'll feature as fascial connection for muscle strolling.

In truth, there can be an Adductor magnus muscle among the two muscle tissues that breaks the relationship.

In this example, it's going to no longer feature as an fascial connection.

2: Muscle routes exchange direction at "stations" of bones and attachments

In the fascial connection, the attachment factors of the muscle businesses that function stations embody bones and tendons that hook up with the bones.

In the muscle instance, the beginning region of the hamstrings is the ischial tuberosity, but on the identical time some of the myofascial fibers at the inspiration of the hamstrings hold from the higher sacral ligament to the sacral vicinity.

As a famous anatomy, the ischial tuberosity is the right answer whilst looking at the muscle by myself, but from the mind-set of "transmission of muscle tension" as fascial connection, the sacral ligament and sacrum also are covered.

The muscle tension as an fascial connection is transmitted to the complete frame by means of the superficial fibers connected to the sacrococcygeal ligament in desire to the deep fibers immediately connected to the bone.

There are also instances wherein a couple of fascial connections are associated from one muscle attachment.

For instance, the rhomboid muscle connected to the scapula extends from the spinous approach of the spinal column to the medial edge of the scapula.

From the medial edge of the scapula, there are styles following the rhomboid muscle, one is the serratus anterior muscle, which connects the scapula to the thorax, and the alternative is the infraspinatus muscle, which connects the scapula to the humerus.

This is likewise a switch that changes the route inside the fascial connection, and connects to the rhomboid muscle, the serratus anterior muscle, and the infraspinatus muscle.

After that, the fascial connection that acts relies upon on the arrangement of the higher limbs and trunk.

This is due to the fact the muscle connection detail thru the bone, that could be a transfer, frequently has multiple muscle mass related to it, and it is pulled from severa commands as a result, and the path of anxiety adjustments relying on the posture of the frame.

By the manner, the serratus anterior is hooked up to the spiral fascia, and the infraspinatus is installation to the fascia at the posterior floor of

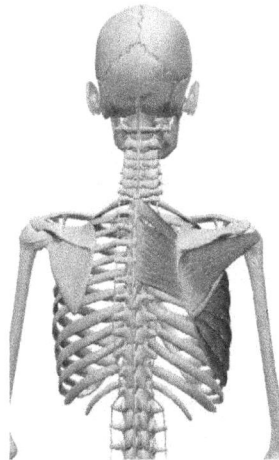

the higher limb.

This is an picture of the rhomboid muscle, infraspinatus muscle, and serratus anterior muscle at the proper side as visible from the lower again.

The rhomboid muscle is within the scapula, the infraspinatus muscle covers the scapula, and the serratus anterior muscle is mounted to the ribs.

These have one-of-a-kind traces that feature relying on the posture in keeping with the policies of the fascial connection.

Express trains and regular trains

The fascial connection expresses the motion of the fascia at the entire frame thru trains and railroad tracks.

The unique teach here is a biarticular muscle that straddles a couple of joints, and the everyday teach is a single joint muscle that straddles exceptional one joint.

In hamstrings, the prolonged head of the biceps femoris extends from the ischial tuberosity to the fibula head and straddles the two joints of the hip and knee joints, as a result acting on these two joints.

On the possibility hand, the brachycephaly of the biceps femoris begins offevolved from the diaphysis of the femur and attaches to the fibula head, so it straddles first-class the knee joint, so it acts on most effective one joint.

The lengthy head of the biceps femoris represents an express educate, and the fast head represents a normal educate.

What is vital proper right here is that it is the biarticular muscular tissues of the everyday train that are extra concerned inside the posture of the body than the biarticular muscle mass of the specific teach.

If the hip joint is confined from stretching or the pelvis is tilted in advance, it's far more powerful to loosen the iliopsoas and pectineus muscle mass, which might be monoarticular muscle mass, than to loosen the rectus femoris muscle tissues of the biarticular muscular tissues.

Chapter 7: Spiral Line(Spl)

Here, we're capable of contact on Spiral Line (SPL).

The SPL wraps in the course of the frame in a spiral that intersects the back and front of the body.

Start from the occipital bone to the shoulders, then through the contralateral ribs and stomach, once more to the unique aspect and via the hip joint.

From the hip joint, it passes from the lateral thigh ⇒ from the front of the decrease leg to the most effective of the foot, and from the fibularis muscle on the lateral aspect of the decrease leg to the hamstrings on the posterior ground of the thigh.

From the ischium, thru the erector spinae muscle groups, the occipital bone, again to the original start.

As a characteristic in the posture of SPL, it runs throughout the frame and has the function of keeping the general balance of the frame.

SPL connects the arch of the best to the pelvis and is worried in knee stability at some stage in movements together with strolling.

When the SPL is shortened or malfunctions, the body twists and tilts to the facet.

Anatomy trains associated with SPL embody SBL, SFL, LL, and DBAL (Deep Back Arm Line).

Due to its large connection, SPL disease moreover influences exquisite anatomy trains.

The left and proper aspects of the SPL are related at the equal time as intersecting, and there can be a distinction in a manner to use the frame like there are right-surpassed and left-surpassed people.

Therefore, it is uncommon that the SPL is perfectly balanced at the left and right.

The motor characteristic of SPL is to purpose a twisting motion (rotation) throughout the frame. It is also associated with the stability of the lower limbs and trunk because of the motion via rotation.

SPL is associated with many awesome anatomy trains.

This moreover method that the lines that make up the SPL make up specific traces at the equal time.

The biceps femoris and erector spinae muscular tissues make up the SBL, and the tibialis anterior and rectus abdominis muscle mass make up the SFL.

The splenius muscle tissue, tensor fasciae latae muscle, and fibula muscle are LL, the rhomboid muscle is DFAL, and the belly muscle agency is FL (Functional Line).

The consequences of SPL on posture embody the pronation and supination of the ankle joint, the rotation of the knee joint, and the rotation of the pelvis as visible from the foot.

Others encompass thoracic rotation with admire to the pelvis, shoulder elevation and anterior deviation, and head tilt and rotation.

Let's take a look at the "stations" and "railroad tracks" of SPL.

Stations here communicate over with bones, and railroad tracks discuss with muscles and fascia. (Notation is from foot to transport)

1: Occipital ridge, mastoid approach, second cervical vertebra (station)

2: Splenius capitis muscle, splenius cervicis muscle (railroad track)

3: Spinous techniques of the decrease cervical spine and better thoracic backbone (station)

four: Rhomboid essential muscle, Rhomboid minor muscle (railroad music)

5: Inner edge of the scapula (station)

6: Serratus anterior (railroad music)

7: Outer part of the ribs (station)

8: External indirect muscle (railroad music)

nine: Abdominal aponeurosis (station)

10: Internal oblique muscle (railroad song)

eleven: Iliac crest, anterior advanced iliac backbone (station)

12: Tensor fasciae latae muscle, iliotibial band (railroad song)

thirteen: Lateral condyle of tibia (station)

14: Tibialis anterior muscle (railroad music)

15: First metatarsal bone base (station)

16: Peroneus longus muscle (railroad music)

17: Fibula head (station)

18: Biceps femoris (railroad song)

19: Ischial tuberosity (station)

20: sacrotuberous ligament (railroad tune)

21: Sacrum (station)

22: Sacral fascia, erector spinae muscle (railroad track)

23: Occipital bone (station)

This is an image of the SPL taken into consideration from the the the front.

The image is the splenius muscle ⇒ rhomboid muscle ⇒ serratus anterior muscle ⇒ oblique muscle enterprise organisation ⇒ tensor fasciae latae muscle.

It moreover represents the biceps femoris, which returns past the lower leg.

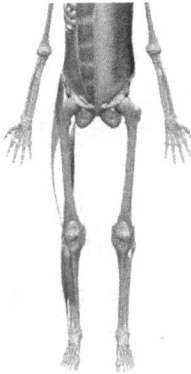

This is an image of the SPL regarded from the front. The image indicates the connection from the oblique muscle ⇒ tensor fasciae latae ⇒ tibialis anterior ⇒ Peroneal ⇒ biceps femoris.

This is an image of the SPL seen from the rear.

You can see the rhomboid muscle businesses, serratus anterior muscle groups, and erector spinae muscle tissues which can be hidden within the picture seen from the the the front.

This is an photograph of the entire SPL.

Chapter 8: Head And Neck

SPL starts offevolved with the occipital crest and mastoid device, becomes the splenius capitis and splenius cervicis muscle agencies, and connects to the spinous strategies of the lower cervical spine and top thoracic spine.

The splenius capitis muscle is likewise the muscle of LL and is related to lateral stability.

The SPL and LL, the splenius capitis muscle and the sternocleidomastoid muscle, function to help the top and neck, and a few ALs furthermore achieve this.

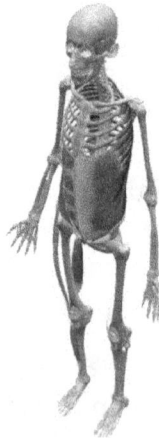

It is the levator scapula muscle that runs from the cervical backbone / thoracic spine to the scapula, and runs parallel to the splenius muscle.

It is much like the rhomboid muscle brought underneath.

It is a extremely good function to assist beforehand traction of the top, but the disadvantage is that the scapula, it truely is the prevent of the muscle, is an risky base.

If this happens, the scapula, that is the bottom of the neck, might be pulled within the course of the neck just so it does not move too an extended manner forward, which may also cause symptoms in the levator scapula muscle.

A comparable case is the trapezius muscle, which additionally has a scapula at the prevent.

When AL compensates for head and neck stability, the scapula turns into pulled up, resulting in impeded arm movement and an inefficient assist sample.

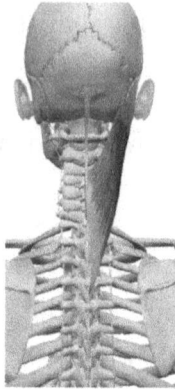

This is an photo of the splenius capitis muscle on the proper factor visible from the lower again.

It originates from the spinous manner of the third thoracic vertebra from the 7th cervical vertebra and is hooked up to the mastoid method of the temporal bone and the occipital bone.

 Its position is to extend the neck, bend laterally, and rotate in the identical direction because the muscle organizations.

This is an photograph of the splenius cervicis muscle on the proper facet seen from the again.

It originates from the spinous strategies of the 0.33 to sixth thoracic vertebrae and attaches to the transverse strategies of the first to one/three cervical vertebrae.

Roles consist of extension of the neck and backbone, lateral flexion, and rotation to the same aspect due to the fact the muscular tissues.

Head and neck launch

To launch the splenius capitis muscle, first ask the trouble to be within the supine function.

 The therapist allows the lower returned of the top from below with one hand.

Place your other hand at the neck of the splenius capitis muscle at the element to be handled. Pinch the tissues proper now above and under the occipital ridge along side your fingertips and flow into them in the direction of the midline.

At that point, the problem should rotate his head toward the component being treated.

Alternatively, the difficulty want to be in a lateral decubitus characteristic, with the hands resting at the hips and the lower once more of the hand touching the pelvis (internal rotation of the better arm and pronation of the hand).

Make positive that the shoulder joint does now not waft due to inner rotation.

The therapist moves his palms to and fro from the acromion to the neck. Alternatively, increase your palms in the course of your shoulders, pulling your ears and shoulders aside, scooping up alongside the anterior fringe of the trapezius muscle.

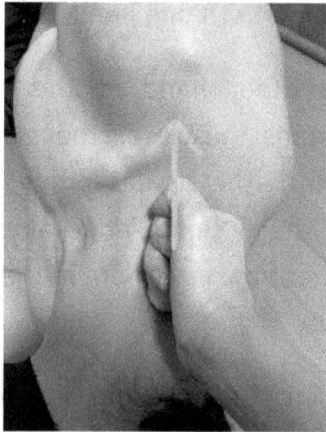

This is an photo of the lateral decubitus role managing the left component (decrease proper is the pinnacle thing). The therapist moves his fingers from the acromion of the shoulder to the neck, spreading from the element to the front and back.

The muscles of the neck can be launched with the useful useful resource of placing a lightly grasped fist from the difficulty's neck to the shoulder and shifting it to scoop up the fist.

Chapter 9: Rhomboid Muscle-Serratus Anterior Muscle

Rhomboid and serratus anterior muscular tissues are muscle groups that have a propensity to motive postural imbalance.

One of the posture collapses because of those muscular tissues is that the scapula is pulled far from the spinal column thru stretching and solving the rhomboid muscle and shortening and solving the serratus anterior muscle.

This is a pattern that has a bent to get up at the same time as your decrease once more is curled up.

In this case, it's far important to boom the serratus anterior muscle just so the rhomboid muscle returns to its precise role.

On the alternative, there may be additionally a sample wherein the rhomboid muscle is shortened and glued, and the serratus anterior muscle is stretched and stuck.

At this time, the medial edge of the scapula is within the course of the spinal column.

In this example, you want to stretch the rhomboid muscular tissues to preserve the scapula away from the spinal column.

This is an photo of the rhomboid muscle on the

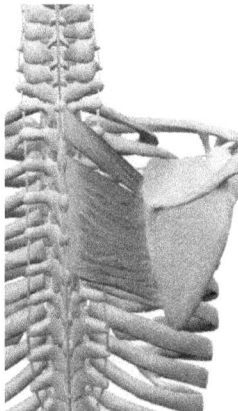

proper trouble seen from the once more.

It is split into , the skinny muscle on the pinnacle is the rhomboid minor muscle, and the thick muscle at the lowest is the rhomboid important muscle.

It originates from the spinous approach of the fifth thoracic vertebra from the seventh cervical vertebra and attaches to the medial edge of the scapula.

Its role is to tug the scapula backwards, rotate the shoulders downwards, pull up the scapulas, stabilize the scapulas, and so on.

This is an photograph of the serratus anterior

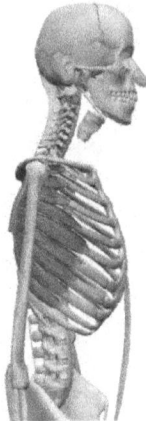

muscle on the right facet as visible from the proper issue.

A muscle that originates from the primary to 9th ribs and attaches to the medial fringe of the scapula.

Its position is to lower the scapula, flip it beforehand, flip the shoulder joint upward, and stabilize the scapula.

Release of rhomboid and serratus anterior muscles

To launch the rhomboid muscle groups, the situation sits in a chair or is in the inclined characteristic, and the therapist places his finger on the spinal column.

From there, float your finger within the course of the shoulder to be treated, pulling the scapula away to the medial fringe of the scapula.

You can use your elbows as opposed to your fingers.

Let's bypass it with the image of pulling it faraway from the spinal column in the direction of the scapula.

To launch the serratus anterior muscle, ask the trouble to take a seat down on a chair or the like.

The therapist stands inside the decrease lower back of and places a gently grasped fist on the outdoor of the trouble's scapula, in the course of the Inferior mind-set.

At this time, the therapist want to vicinity the body as near as viable. By doing so, you could address with less stress.

Have the problem inhale with the attention of pulling up the sternum, and pass the fist closer to the center of the another time because of this.

Move your palms alongside the edges of the scapula. The tissue for your again is pulled down and your chest is pulled up.

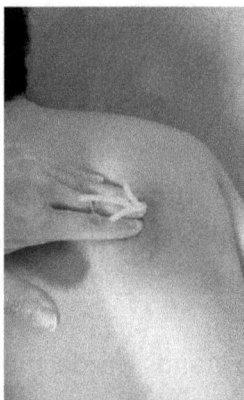

This is an image of the rhomboid muscle being released on the medial edge of the right scapula.

Place your finger from the lower part of the cervical backbone to the higher part of the thoracic backbone to the medial edge of the

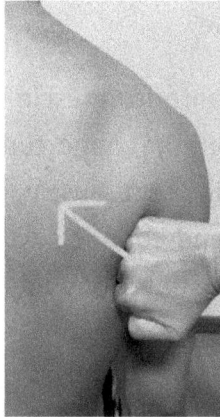

scapula, and flow into your finger to stretch it.

This is an picture of releasing the serratus anterior muscle at the right factor.

Actually, do it with every arms, region your palms alongside the ribs from the outer fringe of the scapula to the lower part of the Inferior mindset, and pass your fist to the spinal column.

External stomach indirect muscle, inner oblique muscle

Rhomboid muscle ⇒ The serratus anterior muscle is strongly associated with the outside indirect muscle.

The serratus anterior muscle ⇒ passes through the thorax on the opportunity factor of the belly outside indirect muscle, crosses the center of the belly, and connects to the inner oblique muscle and the anterior superior iliac backbone on the other thing.

The anterior advanced iliac backbone has many muscular tissues along with the indirect belly muscle, the transverse belly muscle, the tensor fasciae latae muscle, the iliacus muscle, and the sartorius muscle, and pulls them in each route.

In the anatomy educate, it acts like a turntable that switches tracks in every course.

SPL, LL, DFL and SFL are worried as folks who connect with the anterior superior iliac backbone and its surroundings and function an impact on anxiety within the anterior floor of the pelvis.

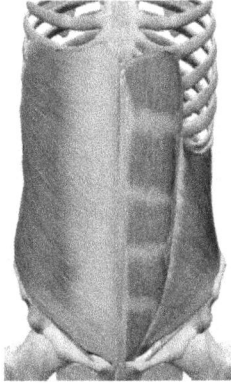

The balance of each anatomy train keeps the region and tilt of the pelvis.

It is an photograph of the out of doors oblique muscle at the right aspect, the rectus abdominis muscle at the left aspect, and the internal indirect muscle.

These deep layers have transversus abdominis muscle tissue. In the photograph, the rectus abdominis and indirect muscle mass are separated, however in terms of fascia, they may be included with the useful resource of the fascia of the indirect and transverse belly muscle tissue as they descend from the starting vicinity of the fifth rib. Layers skip from shallow to deep.

The roles of the External oblique and internal indirect include flexion, lateral flexion, and rotation of the trunk.

Release of the outside indirect and inner oblique muscle groups

Release from the muscle of the anterior superior iliac spine.

The state of affairs is within the supine feature and the therapist hooks his finger at the aponeurosis of the abdomen along the iliac crest.

From there, bypass your palms all through the stomach muscles inward and upward in the stomach.

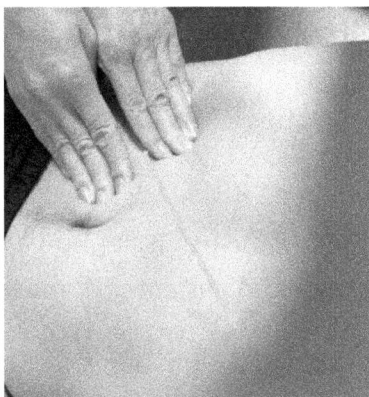

Move your hand past the middle of the stomach until you reach the opposite chest, and then to the outdoor of the chest wherein the serratus anterior muscle companies are located.

This is an image of the oblique muscle agencies released inside the SPL on the proper. Move your finger from the anterior superior iliac backbone to the contralateral thorax.

iliotibial band

At the bottom of the SPL, the anatomy educate runs in a huge circle from the hip joint to the foot.

The internal indirect muscle connects to the iliac crest and the anterior superior iliac backbone, from which it connects to the tensor fasciae latae muscle.

In LL, it connects from the tensor fasciae latae muscle to the fibula muscle, however in SPL it connects to the tibialis anterior muscle.

The SPL connects the tensor fasciae latae muscle to the iliotibial band, which has a big band of tissue on the outdoor of the thigh this is with out troubles handy.

The iliotibial band is placed on the surface of the vastus lateralis muscle and expands from the knee to the hip joint.

By the time it reaches the hip joint, it covers the out of doors of the hip joint with the iliotibial band, the tensor fasciae latae muscle, the deep gluteus medius muscle, and the top fibers of the posterior gluteus maximus muscle.

When the iliotibial band becomes traumatic, the pelvis is pulled ultimately, inflicting lateral movement and tilting of the pelvis.

In addition, the imbalance a number of the iliotibial band and the adductor muscular tissues of the hip joint can cause O-legs and X-legs.

This is an image of the tensor fasciae latae muscle on the right issue and the iliotibial band visible from the the front proper aspect.

It originates from the iliac crest and the anterior superior iliac backbone and connects to the iliotibial band.

Roles embody hip flexion, abduction, and internal rotation.

Release across the iliotibial band

To release the location for the duration of the iliotibial band, first ask the priority to stand left or right and be in a lateral decubitus function.

The therapist facilitates the knee of the higher leg and applies a gently grasped fist to the muscle tissues related to the iliotibial band (tensor fasciae latae, gluteus maximus, gluteus medius).

Move your hands to unfold out of the iliotibial band.

Alternatively, the therapist can launch the iliotibial band via way of setting the forearm simply underneath the iliac crest and shifting the elbow down within the course of the problem's knee.

By adjusting the angle of the forearm, the therapist can adjust the a part of the iliotibial band that he / she wants to launch if there may be a tough aspect inside the anterior or posterior component.

It is also possible to use the therapist's elbow to region it throughout the extra trochanter of the problem and launch the muscle groups inside the course of the better part of the pelvis which includes the iliac crest and iliac spine.

the therapist can launch the iliotibial band by manner of placing the forearm truly under the iliac crest and shifting the elbow down in the direction of the scenario's knee.

The tensor fasciae latae muscle and gluteal muscle organization may be released with the aid of utilising pressure to the location from the greater trochanter to the iliac crest with the elbow.

Chapter 10: Lower Leg The Front

The Lateral condyle of tibia connects to the tibialis anterior muscle.

The anterior part of the decrease leg includes the tibialis anterior muscle, the extensor digitorum longus muscle, and the extensor hallucis longus muscle, which shape the anterior compartment of the lower leg.

The tibialis anterior muscle runs from the knee inward and inferiorly all of the way all of the manner right down to the foot and attaches to the medial cuneiform bone of the tarsal bone and the primary metatarsal bone. Fascial connections to the peroneus longus may be seen at the soles of the feet.

In addition, the muscle of the lower leg front might be controlled movement through the extensor retinaculum at the ankle. With the extensor retinaculum, the muscle tendon is regular to the ankle and acts as a pulley to exert stress successfully.

If the pressure from the extensor retinaculum is robust, the muscle tissue inside the the front of the decrease leg may not slide easily and the motion of the ankle joint can be restrained, or the decrease limbs may be in a in advance leaning posture.

Anterior tilt of the decrease limbs is a scenario wherein the knee joint protrudes in the the front of the ankle joint, the gastrocnemius muscle of the calf is stretched, and the muscle groups in the front of the decrease leg consisting of the tibialis anterior muscle are attracted downward.

This is a the front view of the tibialis anterior muscle at the right component.

It originates from the lateral condyle of the tibia and the proximal bone frame, passes thru the anterior surface of the decrease leg, and attaches to the number one metatarsal bone and the medial cuneiform bone.

Roles consist of dorsiflexion and varus of the ankle.

Release of the the the front of the lower leg

Ask the priority to be in the supine characteristic and perform plantar dorsiflexion of the ankle joint at the difficulty to be handled.

At this time, do now not carry out distinct moves which include varus or valgus of the ankle joint.

The therapist gently grasps the fist and locations it beneath the extensor retinaculum on the another time of the foot, and makes use of the alternative hand to sell the trouble's ankle plantar dorsiflexion.

While transferring your legs, pull your fist up from the extensor retinaculum at the identical time as applying stress to the tibia.

If the hardness of the extensor retinaculum limits the gliding homes of the ankle dorsiflexor muscle mass, the discharge of these can enhance the mobility of the ankle joint.

Alternatively, the therapist uses each arms to method the tibialis anterior muscle and tibia.

At this time, the therapist locations a gently grasped fist (MP joint) on the challenge's extensor retinaculum, on the tibia and tibialis anterior muscle groups.

Make high quality that the joint within the center of the finger (PIP joint) faces each special with each arms, and exercise pressure to the hand located on the tibia just so it does no longer cause pain.

The difficulty is requested to bend the ankle joint within the equal way as earlier than, and the therapist increases the hand in keeping with the dorsiflexion of the foot and prevents the hand in the case of plantar flexion.

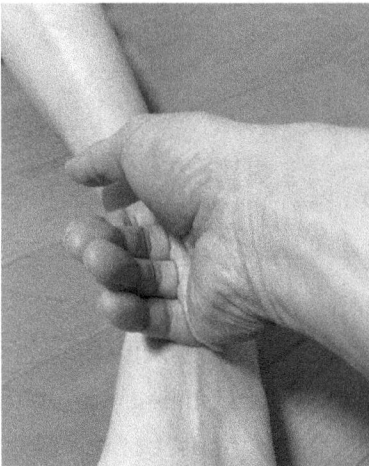

Let's do that gadget as masses due to the fact the pinnacle of the tibia.

This is an image of releasing the extensor retinaculum on the decrease again of the foot.

Place a lightly grasped fist at the distal cease of the ankle and raise the fist over the ankle whilst having the challenge bend the ankle.

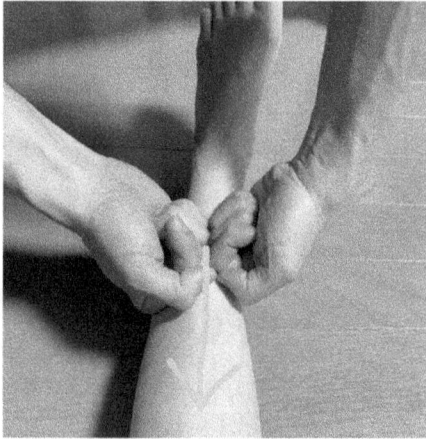

This is an photo of treating the tibialis anterior muscle and tibia with each fingers. While combined fist, we're pulling up within the direction of the better aspect of the tibia.

When you attain the pinnacle of the tibia, open your fists to spread them inward and outward.

Side of lower leg

The sole of the foot connects the metatarsal bones to the fibula muscle businesses.

The peroneus longus and peroneus brevis are fused due to the fact the vastus lateralis septum. The decrease leg has multiple muscle tissue separated thru fascia.

For example, the gastrocnemius and soleus muscle mass are inside the superficial posterior compartment, the posterior tibial muscle and flexor digitorum longus are inside the deep posterior compartment, and the tibialis anterior and prolonged and quick toe extensor muscle mass are in the anterior compartment.

If you waft up the fibula from the outer ankle and hint the fibula under the muscular tissues, you can divide it into anterior compartment and lateral compartment.

When the ankle joint is dorsiflexed, you can sense the difference inside the part of the muscle contraction within the vastus lateralis septum.

The muscle tissues of the anterior compartment

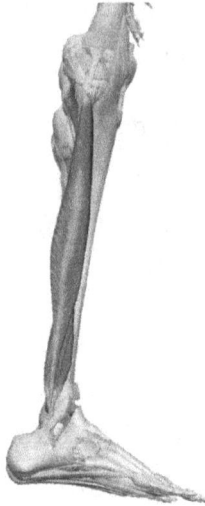

act throughout dorsiflexion, and the muscle groups of the posterior compartment act in some unspecified time in the future of plantar flexion.

The peroneus brevis originates from the diaphysis of the fibula, whilst the peroneus longus originates from the peroneus head, it actually is the higher stop of the fibula.

This is an image of the fibula muscle at the proper facet as seen from the proper issue.

The fibularis muscle is often used to save you dorsiflexion of the ankle joint in the repute feature, and shortening of the fibularis muscle reasons valgus of the ankle joint.

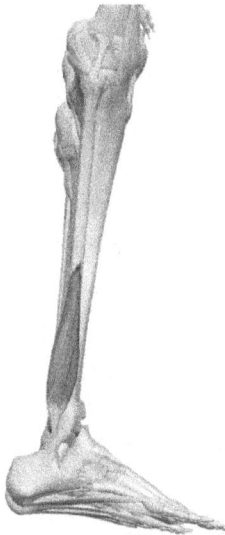

The peroneus longus muscle originates from the top 2/3 of the diaphysis of the fibula and attaches to the first metatarsal bone and the medial cuneiform bone.

The peroneus brevis muscle originates from the decrease 2/3 of the peroneus diaphysis and attaches to the 5th metatarsal bone.

Its actions encompass raising the heel (plantar flexion) and turning the most effective of the foot outward (valgus).

This is an photograph of the peroneus longus muscle at the proper component as seen from the right thing.

This is an photograph of the peroneus brevis muscle at the right issue as visible from the proper factor. The peroneus brevis is deep in the peroneus longus.

Release of the component of the decrease leg

Ask the hassle to be inside the lateral decubitus function.

It is a amazing idea to region a cushion a few of the assignment's feet because it will positioned pressure on the decrease legs.

We will release the fibula muscle tissues alongside the fibula, but one method is to area the therapist's finger alongside the fibula and stretch it to and fro at some point of the fibula.

While doing this, permit the priority bend the ankle joint and drift the hand toward the foot.

There is also a way to method the entire fascia of the lower leg in preference to the fibula muscle.

For example, on the same time because the ankle joint is supination, the SPL, the fibula muscle, is pulled down and the medial part of the decrease leg is lifted.

In this example, in place of coming near the leg muscle agencies in my opinion, flow your arms to stretch the fascia on the medial and lateral elements of the lower leg.

If the ankle is supination, to address it, vicinity a gently gripped fist on the inside and outside of the lower leg, pull the inner hand down towards the ankle, and pull the outer hand up towards the knee.

At this time, make sure that each fingers are going via every wonderful to a degree and now

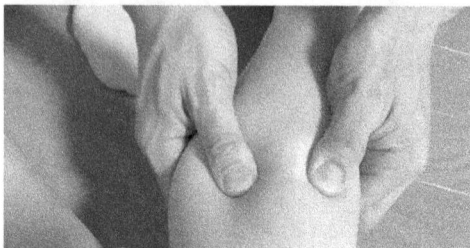

not too a ways aside.

Touch the fibula from the out of doors of the lower leg and use your hands to stretch the fibula muscle organizations connected to the fibula within the anterior-posterior course.

At this time, ask the scenario to bend the ankle joint dorsiflexion.

Place your fist gently toward the fibula head and pull your fist down towards your foot.

Place your fists at the inside and outside of your decrease legs. If the ankle is turned around, pull the outer (fibularis aspect) fist up and the internal fist down.

Posterior thigh

In the SPL, the fibula muscle connects to the fibula head, then the lateral hamstrings, the biceps femoris, to the ischial tuberosity.

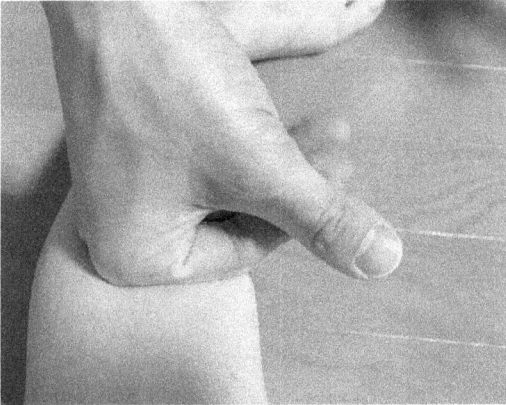

Hamstrings have semitendinosus, semimembranosus, and biceps femoris, however except for the brachycephaly of the biceps femoris, they may be unique educate muscle tissues that straddle the hip and knee joints.

Hamstrings are divided into lateral and medial, with the lateral biceps femoris and the medial semitendinosus and semimembranosus.

Actions embody hip extension and knee flexion.

The distinction a number of the medial and lateral is that the medial hamstrings rotate the knee (tibia) internally and the lateral hamstrings rotate the knee externally.

These movements are often applied in sports sports sports situations which includes strenuous movements.

To see if the hamstrings are operating one by one at the medial and lateral components, place your knees in the inclined feature along aspect your knees bent and call upwards from the popliteal fossa.

Move your finger closer to the ischial tuberosity, placing aside the internal and outer hamstrings.

Generally, about 10 cm above the popliteal fossa, the medial and lateral hamstrings meet.

You also can see if muscle contraction is taking place with the resource of manner of twisting your legs inward or outward (inner or outdoor rotation) collectively with your knees bent.

Two strains of regular trains run deep in the biceps femoris, it truely is an explicit teach.

One of them is the brachycephaly of the biceps femoris, which extends from the Linea aspera of the femur (diaphysis) to the fibula head.

If the knee is chronically bent or the tibia is externally turned round, the biceps femoris brachycephaly can be shortened or the anxiety may be extended.

The one-of-a-type muscle is the adductor muscle, which extends from the ischium to the decrease a part of the pubis, the Linea aspera of the femur, and the medial epicondyle.

Shortening and improved anxiety motive the pelvis to tilt backwards, that is a component that hinders hip movement.

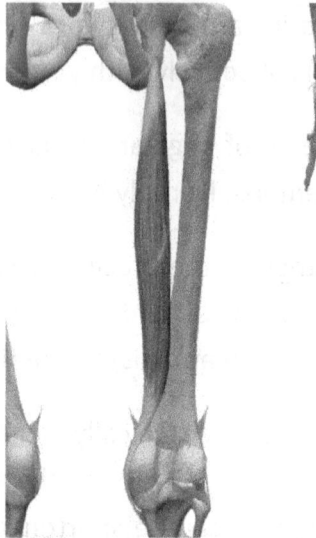

This is an picture of the semitendinosus muscle, which is the medial hamstrings of the proper leg, visible from the again.

It originates from the ischial tuberosity and attaches to the pes anserinus on the medial anterior ground of the tibia.

The roles consist of knee flexion, internal rotation, hip extension, and inner rotation.

It is a biarticular muscle that straddles the hip and knee joints.

This is an photograph of the semimembranosus muscle, that is the medial hamstrings of the proper leg, visible from the lower once more.

It originates from the ischial tuberosity and attaches to the medial condyle of the tibia.

Its role is to flex the knee joint, inner rotation, hip extension, and inner rotation further to the semitendinosus muscle.

It is a biarticular muscle that straddles the hip

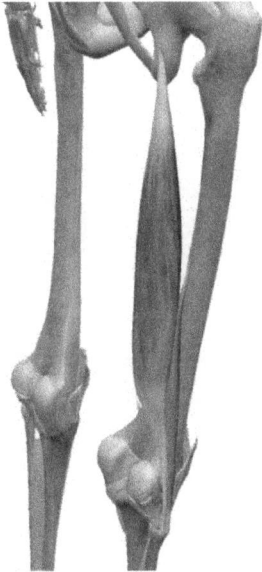

and knee joints.

This is an photograph of the biceps femoris (long head / short head), it's the outer hamstrings on the proper thing.

The extended head originates from the ischial tuberosity and the fast head originates from the Linea aspera at the posterior ground of the femur and extends past the knee to the fibula head.

The roles consist of flexion of the knee joint, outdoor rotation, extension of the hip joint, and external rotation.

Chapter 11: Release Of The Posterior Thigh

It may be a launch of the entire hamstrings in place of the biceps femoris.

Ask the hassle to be within the inclined position and maintain the knee bent ninety ranges. The therapist holds the foot down and stabilizes it.

Ask the situation to stretch their knees step by step, with their palms putting aside the internal and outer hamstrings of the yet again of the knee.

Hand addressed to the hamstrings will maintain to place the strain if you want to boom the inner out of doors the tendon.

To launch the hamstrings, region your hands on the edges of the medial and lateral hamstrings and have the scenario bend and stretch their knees to release the muscle tissues.

When treating best to the biceps femoris, the trouble must be in a lateral decubitus feature with the leg to be handled going through up.

Bend your legs forward and solid them with cushions.

The therapist places his finger at the stomach of the biceps femoris close to the trailing edge of the iliotibial band and stretches the tissue towards the knee.

You can stretch your muscular tissues more by

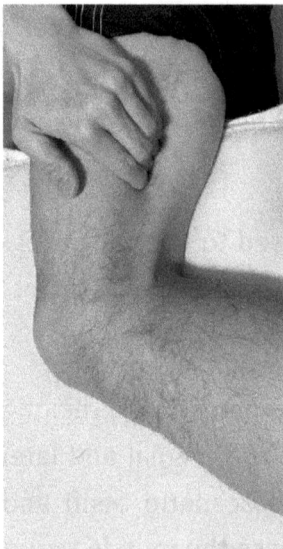

using stretching your knees lightly.

This is an image of the proper thigh visible from the out of doors.

Place your finger at the trailing edge of the iliotibial band and the biceps femoris to growth it.

As you method your knees, you can touch the brachycephaly of your biceps femoris.

Back

There is an erector spinae muscle that ascends from the lateral hamstrings and connects to the Sacrotuberous ligament.

There are shallow explicit trains collectively with the longissimus and iliocostalis muscle tissues, deep normal trains which incorporates the spinalis, semispinalis and multifidus muscle companies, and the intertransversarii muscle groups inside the deeper layers. This is likewise an SBL on the aspect of the hamstrings.

The superficial muscle tissue of the explicit train are SBL and on the same time associated with the surrounding muscle groups such as the splenius muscle, rhomboid muscle, levator scapula muscle, trapezius muscle, and latissimus dorsi muscle.

The above muscle tissue make up the SPL, Arm Line (AR), and Functional Line (FL), which additionally have an impact on every exceptional with different myofascial meridians.

To recognize the nation of the spinal column, we are able to first have a look at the curve of the spine.

Look at the anterior curvature of the cervical and lumbar vertebrae, the posterior curvature of the thoracic vertebrae, whether or not the spinous techniques are raised like mountains, and whether or not or no longer the depressions close to the spinous techniques are

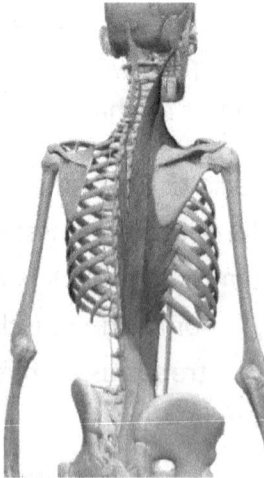

like valleys.

This is an photo of the erector spinae muscle corporations on the proper component seen from the decrease decrease lower back.

From the inner of the spinal column, the spinalis, longissimus, and iliocostalis muscle corporations. Roles include trunk extension and lateral bending.

This is an image of the semispinalis and multifidus muscle corporations on the proper component as visible from the again. The first rate muscle groups that run above the thorax are the semispinalis, and the band-shaped muscle corporations underneath the thorax are the multifidus muscle agencies. The roles of the semispinalis are trunk extension, lateral flexion and rotation, and the multifidus muscle is trunk extension and rotation, and spinal balance.

This is an image of the rotatores and intertransversarii muscle groups at the proper difficulty as visible from the rear.

The rotatores run diagonally from the transverse technique to the spinous method above the thorax, and the intertransversarii muscle companies run narrowly on the rims of

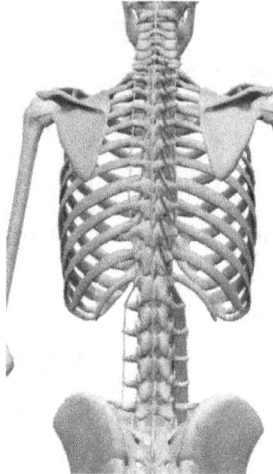

the lumbar spine and the transverse method of the thorax.

 The deeper the muscle, the more it's miles connected as a unmarried joint.

Release of the lower once more

To launch the erector spinae muscle tissues, first ask the problem to take a seat down down in a chair with their feet at the floor after which straighten their backs and appearance proper away in advance.

Looking at the location of the spinous manner and the surrounding muscles, it looks as if a mountain while the spinous gadget is better than the surroundings, and a valley at the identical time as it's miles buried as compared to the surrounding muscle tissues.

At this time, pull the chin definitely so the once more neck extends.

From there, the trunk is bent beforehand with the image of transferring the spine one at a time.

The therapist seems at the motion of the backbone and reveals out in which the movements of the spinous tactics are separated separately and become immobile.

The therapist stands in the decrease returned of the difficulty and places his hand at the region of the spine that isn't always shifting.

At this time, gently draw close the fist and location the proximal phalanx of the finger on each elements of the problem's spine.

As the hassle starts to bend, the therapist pulls his fist down, pushing it inward or outward in opposition to the spine.

In the case of mountains, circulate your palms in the direction of the spinous strategies, and within the case of valleys, flow your hands in order that they spread outward toward the encompassing muscle tissue.

When the spinous machine is excessive, the encircling muscles are frequently widened, so bypass it closer to the mountain spinous device.

When the spinous processes are sinking, the encompassing muscle groups are too close to every extraordinary, so unfold them apart. Therapist might be can be finished wherein include the elbow in region of the fist.

Treatment is viable even in a susceptible position. At that time, the therapist places the fist at the state of affairs's spine.

At this time, make an opening collectively together with your fist so as now not to apply strain to the spinous method.

SPL stretch

SPL is concerned in twisting moves of the body. For instance, the motion of attaching one elbow to the alternative knee (crunch) makes use of the better muscle mass of the SPL.

There are the following due to the fact you may stretch in particular with the aid of together with a twisting movement along with the trunk.

• The triangular pose in yoga stretches the higher SPL, at the same time as some SPLs show muscle contraction to hold posture.

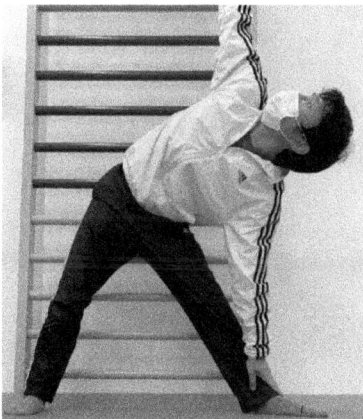

• Sit on the floor together along with your legs extended, bend one knee and vicinity your legs outdoor the opportunity leg. You can stretch the higher SPL with the aid of twisting your higher frame to the aspect in which your knees are bent. It is normally executed as a stretch on the buttocks and the outdoor of the thighs.

This is a triangular pose in yoga. You can mainly stretch the SPL of the trunk and hip joints.

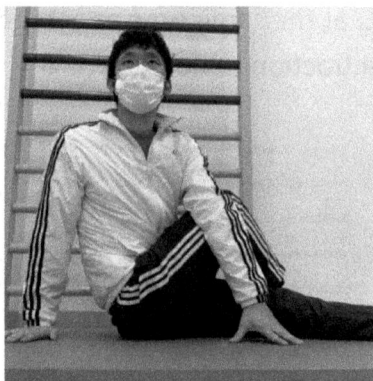

As proven in the picture, you may stretch the SPL of the trunk through the usage of setting one foot on the outside of the alternative leg and twisting the body.

Chapter 12: A Guide To Self Treatment

Trigger elements are normally used by expert therapists, but, they also may be used by humans in order to release anxiety inside the cause factors.

While there are obvious regulations, concerning what we are able to self-launch (despite the whole lot a trained professional, utilizing stress from a strategic mind-set, is going to have extra fulfillment at stepping into hard to obtain regions), masses of physical tensions.

The trouble to go through in mind, however, is that cause points will now not release if we use a namby-pamby approach. If you have got ever been to a bodily therapist, then you may maintain in mind the ache, sure pain is the proper word right here. The degree of consolation felt is essentially proportional to three factors:

1.The willingness of the affected individual to go through pain (even ache)

2.Knowledge of the practitioner

three.The frequency of the remedy

Just bear in mind those 3 elements, for a minute. If we are willing to undergo pain, then a greater level of launch can be felt. But to undergo a horrendous consultation of Self Myofascial Release (SMR), in which a excellent treatment is felt and then simplest to go away the entirety by myself for weeks till the hassle will become chronic all over again, is an entire waste of time. Also, the alternative of that could be a namby-pamby method, in which we go through the motions, however we never truely get the discharge, within the first location, is also a complete waste of our time and effort.

So, the method, which we need to take, is one wherein we are willing to push sufficient to provide a launch (but not always a mind-blowing hour and a half of of of prolonged, sweating, agonising one), but in addition importantly we need to carry out each day durations. Maybe no longer every day durations, of the only body element, maybe break up the body parts over severa intervals, however the concept is to do ten to 20 mins a day often. When we take this approach, grade

146

by grade, we get the comfort which we need, due to the fact the physical imbalances slowly proper themselves.

Another problem, which need to moreover be remembered, is that bodily rubdown isn't sufficient. These physical imbalances typically arose out of way of existence imbalances, over an extended term, and manner of lifestyles changes additionally want to be made. For instance, say you have got were given a soleus hassle collectively with your calf, and have all forms of aches and pains; positive the cause elements will beneficial beneficial aid comfort, but probably you want to trade your footwear, get corrective sole allows to your fallen arches and change some factors of your walking gait, maybe you'll even ought to exchange the manner you're taking a seat down and perform a little different bodily sports activities, which includes Pilates or yoga, for example, and perhaps a few center carrying occasions, in order to rebalance your posture, simplest then will a complete healing take area.

So we ought to suppose in phrases of ten to 20 minutes a day, over a length of months training those SMR strategies, while also running on our numerous imbalances and life-style changes. This might sound severe, as we are residing within the age of "take a pill and forget about approximately it", however significantly in case you need to get everlasting comfort from orthopedic stiffness and ache, the approach to take is absolutely one in all walking through imbalances, over the years. Take this method and splendid results will take area!

Finally, searching at launch over again, we want to be willing to capture and squeeze the muscle and fascia.

Hands

We can use our forefinger, thumb, forefinger and thumb or hand take hold of.

Forefinger:We can use our forefinger to poke round. This is terrific from a diagnostic factor of view, because the right way to discover a motive thing is to poke round until ache is felt, however it's normally missing the critical electricity to result in release.

Thumb:Our thumbs are truly strong, so obviously they're unique at prodding into difficult to achieve places, and gaining treatment.

Forefinger and Thumb:This is a extraordinary mixture, wherein we will hold near the region and observe stress to the motive problem, for fast effective consolation.

Knuckles:Knuckles are a without a doubt high-quality way of getting a deep, sharp, localised

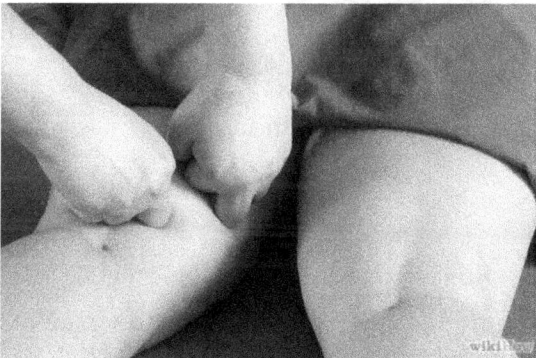

impact into a particular vicinity.

Picture courtesy of wikihow

Hand Grab:This can be a beneficial method, whereby we're capable of benefit even more leverage. A sincerely proper instance of hand take hold of may be accomplished on our higher traps, wherein we reason for the midmost component and take hold of the lure as although were approximately to elevate up a six p.C., however rather we take preserve of, hold and squeeze.

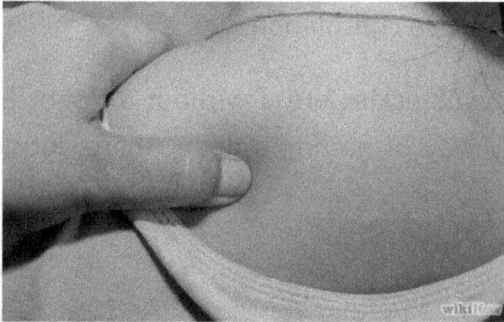

Picture courtesy of wikihow

Tools

Foam Roller:The foam curler might be the maximum famous SMR device, and virtually it is a curler with foam on it!

How do we use it correctly?

Simply discover the reason aspect and roll from side to side over it till launch comes. This is right for huge areas, such as legs, decrease again, better decrease back, hip area and so forth. The secret's to keep rolling and operating closer to getting a tighter squeeze on this location. Once

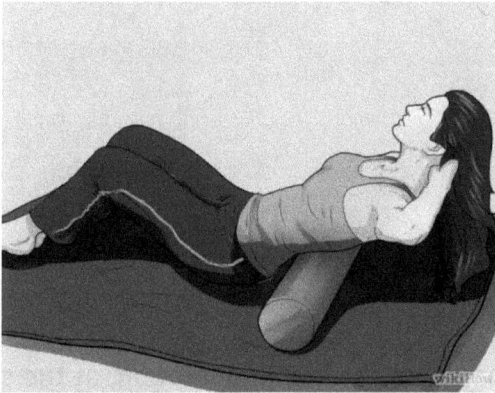

you get into it, a vital feeling of ache and stress will increase and truly have a look at the ache because it slowly releases. Work at it for ten to 15 minutes, from a number of angles after which permit it go till the next day, don't forget Rome emerge as no longer built in an afternoon!

Picture courtesy of wikihow

Massage ball:The massage ball (it doesn't should be a rubdown ball, as any kind of hardball, rubber ball and so on., will do the method), is right for those hard to attain locations, collectively with shoulders, chest, and clearly particular factors of the lower decrease lower back, Think of the foam roller as some

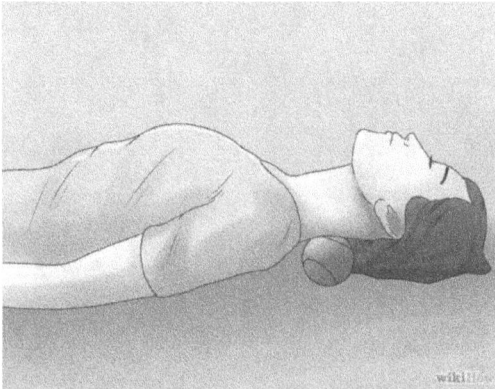

thing large and stupid in operation, at the same time as the ball is small and sharp, so it's a higher device for moving into difficult to achieve places, in which the ache is more localised. In many procedures, its operation is just like knuckle rub down, but obviously, it permits us to get admission to elements of our private frame, which we could not get proper of get right of entry to to via our knuckles.

Picture courtesy of wikihow

Chapter 13: Neck And Head Pain

1. Splenius capitas

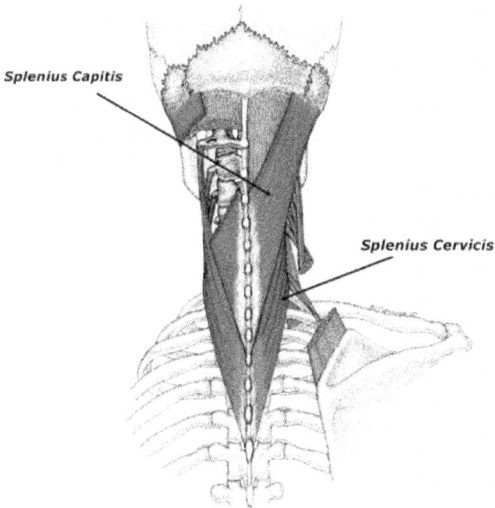

Description:

The splemius capitas is a muscle which runs from the top again and cervical location of the neck upto the pinnacle of the top. The fibers run upwards and outwards and inserts underneath the sternomastoid muscle, into the mastoid manner behind the ear and at the lowest of the skull.

Function:

The characteristic of this muscle is to stabilize the neck, as there are muscle groups each one taking walks along the issue of the neck. These muscle corporations stabilize the neck and help to move the assist the top to move backwards.

Symptoms:

Splenius capitas issues result in ache and throbbing sensations inside the top of the pinnacle. Often sensations of burning or tinkling are also discovered within the top head place.

Trigger Point Therapy:

To launch this issue, really direct pressure onto the relevant thing as visible inside the diagram underneath.

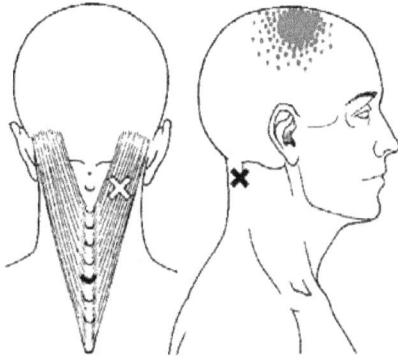

A 2d manner to art work the factor is to stretch it whilst shifting the pinnacle beforehand and a long way from the facet being handled. You can also use a rub or muscle ache spray at the neck place in advance than trying the stretch. Importantly you have that allows you to drift your neck ahead, once more and sideways with out restrict.

If you feel a limit in your neck accompanied through a throbbing pain it is probably that this thing wishes to be released. It's genuinely simply really worth trying to launch the element and then see the manner you get on.

Start out with the aid of the usage of using strain at the point first and if a few release is felt then strive stretching the neck out lightly. Releasing a point with strain may even require a agency press but on the identical time as stretching the neck strive now not to position undue strain on the neck as this will make it worse.

2. Temporalis

Description:

The temporalis is a fan-formed muscle located at the side of the top. It originates on the temporal bone of the cranium and its fibers converge at the jawbone. In easy English the temporalis muscle runs from the facet of the top proper down to the jawbone, truly take a look at the diagram beneath. The temporalis cause factor is found definitely above the temple bone, a bone which runs from the top ear to the attention socket. As the diagram well-knownshows there are four sub-points which all lie along the period of the temporalis muscle tissue and which may be inspired.

Function:

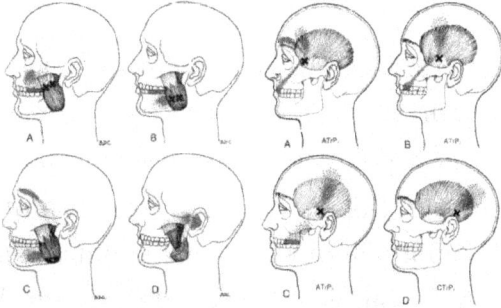

The important feature of the temporalis muscle is to close the mouth. Its upper fiber can be felt above the temple even as the jaw is clenched.

Symptoms:

Various courtroom times may be located in this muscle. Uneven enamel and accidents to the face generally have an impact right here. Also Trigeminal neuralgia (a state of affairs wherein one facet of the face suffers from worrying nerve ache), also can purpose troubles right here. Stress and anxiety also can have an effect at the face. So symptoms and symptoms can range from ache to weird sensations to a modern-day disturbance within the facial location.

Trigger Point Therapy:

The best way to get going with this thing is to press your forefinger towards your cheekbone after which pull your finger lower again closer to your ear. Depending upon the scale of your head, about half of to as a minimum one inch a ways from your ear clearly slide your forefinger up over the cheekbone and then you'll sense the smooth fleshy are which is called the temple.

Now because the diagram suggests there are surely 4 motive points taking walks alongside this muscle, from near the eye after which right once more to an area without a doubt past your ear. The method which has referred to above is a extremely good place to begin. You can then are searching for alongside this line which runs in fact over the cheekbone and hunt down for touchy areas and anywhere you experience a sensitive spot, without a doubt press and keep for approximately twenty seconds or so. Release and repeat for twenty seconds and reap this severa times in advance than moving onto the alternative sub-factors.

Chapter 14: Chest And Back And Shoulders

3. Sternalis

Description:

The sternalis is an area of tissue which covers the sternum (breastplate).

Function:

It has no obvious feature aside from it's a popular piece of fascia and like all fascia, it helps to maintain muscle companies ligaments and tendons in place.

Symptoms:

This is a extraordinary thing for ache in the chest place and particular any kind of chest bone ache.

Trigger Point Therapy:

This point is extra or tons less an intuitive point. Simply hint a line from the begin of the sternum up severa inches until you find the maximum sensitive a part of the sternum and then in reality press for twenty seconds and release,

take a few seconds out and then repeat severa
instances.

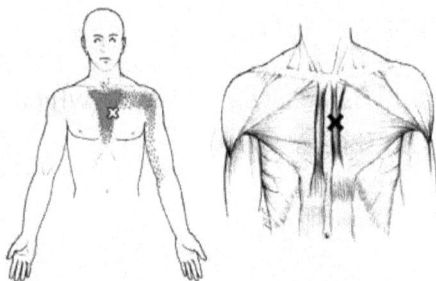

four. Pectoralis major (Sternal Division)

Description:

This is the big triangular a part of the pectoralis
muscle (breast muscle), which runs from the
ribcage as much as the shoulder joint at the
threshold of the pinnacle arm.

Function:

This a part of the pectoralis muscle's
characteristic is to elevate the arm ahead and in
the course of the midline of the body. It
additionally permits to rotate the arm inwards.

Symptoms:

Pain within the chest muscle, specially inside the course of the outer arm and emotions of anxiety. This can get up from going for walks out which include lifting weights or doing push-ups, however additionally tension and pain right right right here can originate because of blunt trauma to the frame, which includes minor or important accidents.

Trigger Point Therapy:

To discover this problem, test the diagram below and then try to maintain close your pectoralis muscle as if you were trying to pinch some difficulty. The thumb ought to be on the pectoralis muscle, at the same time because the forefinger and center palms need to within the place of the armpit. Have a experience round till you find out some tenderness after which work at pressing for twenty seconds and then permit bypass for ten seconds and then repeat numerous instances on this equal factor. You also can have a enjoy round for what are named in Traditional Chinese Medicine as "Local Points", a neighborhood component been everywhere wherein pain and tension is held in the muscle businesses and fascia.

five. Pectoralis main (Clavicular Division)

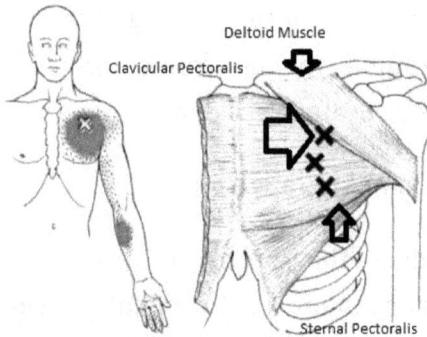

Deltoid Muscle
Clavicular Pectoralis
Sternal Pectoralis

Description:

This a part of the pectoralis muscle runs from the inner half of of of of the collarbone proper proper down to the higher part of the shoulder insertion. This reason factor of the pectoralis is basically barely higher up than sternal section of the pectoralis muscle.

Function:

This muscle enables with bending and raising the pinnacle arm.

Symptoms:

Pain in the breast region radiating out towards the arm and often relates to intellectual-emotional strain.

Trigger Point Therapy:

The manner to distinguish amongst sternal and clavicular pectoralis muscles is to raise your arm after which get someone to forestall you raising your arm above shoulder degree. When you do so, you shall word that the clavicular phase of the pectoralis muscle activates. Whereas the sternal a part of the pectoralis muscle turns on a bargain lower, as we strive and keep our arm out near nipple level.

Where then can we press for motive issue consolation?

Well have a enjoy around close to the very higher part of your pectoralis muscle near the shoulder/pinnacle arm, close to the place have been the deltoid passes over the pectoralis muscle, surely check the photo all over again.

6. Multifidus spinae

Description:

The multifidis spinae are a sequence of strips of muscle groups which run parallel to the backbone from the bottom of the spine proper as plenty because the neck.

Function:

These are postural muscle corporations which control center balance of the spinal joints. They additionally have an effect on side bending and rotating torso movements.

Symptoms:

Pain on this area. The ache might be everywhere, so in area of getting hung up on a particular factor suppose in phrases of capability "close by factors", elements that could shift barely from man or woman to man or woman.

Trigger Point Therapy:

The only manner to get the factors right here is to seize both your waist, if the pain is in this area, and then squeeze together along with your thumb from at the back of and your hands from the front of your torso. If the pain isn't placed near the waist area then ask a helper to revel in across the once more area near the spine and every time you enjoy ache or anxiety, get them to squeeze and release this aspect. Also, stretching additionally can be proper idea here whilst blended with motive points.

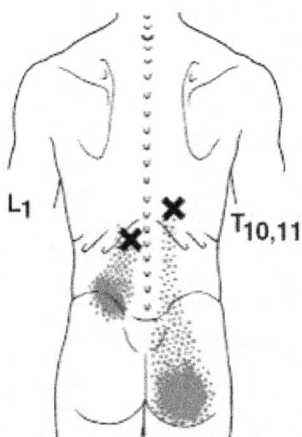

7. Longissimus dorsi

Description:

The longissimus dorsi belong to the erector spinae muscle mass (the muscle mass which lie alongside the lower cease of the once more muscular tissues which help to bend over or stand once more up at the same time as maintaining one's legs right now.)

Function:

These muscle groups help the spine to bend in advance, all over again or sideways.

Symptoms:

Pain everywhere from the 8-rib all of the way proper all the way down to the buttock. The nature of fascia been what it is, the ache can in reality as without problem be nebulous as it is able to be particular.

Trigger Point Therapy:

Feel your lower yet again near your backbone and press the place of ache or sensitivity. Foam rolling can be suitable and moreover a awesome technique is to take both a massage ball (baseball, cricket ball or tough rubber ball will art work without troubles nicely). When the use of a massage ball, place the ball in opposition to the wall and press your lower back in opposition to the ball and squeeze hard, launch and repeat several instances.

Also, do no longer get hung up on one component, as an opportunity experience a sensitive spot and art work on it some instances, then flow into round your once more. Often you'll find that because of the reality the ache releases, that the ache begins offevolved moving round each the lower, mid once more or the buttocks. So revel in your manner through the tension and paintings in the direction of a release.

8. Posterior cervical

Description:

These muscular tissues be part of from the decrease cervical and better thoracic place.

Function:

The cause of these muscle tissues is to assist flow into the pinnacle forwards decrease returned and sideways.

Symptoms:

Pain within the neck, base of the skull or lack of capability to move the neck absolutely.

Trigger Point Therapy:

The posterior cervical muscle mass generally tend to overlap every different, so a certain type of moves can be required to get a tremendous trigger release. Probably palms and thumb are the amazing manner to transport and often a trustworthy quantity of pressure can be required, commonly implemented toward the returned of the neck close to the bottom of the cranium. As continually squeeze for twenty to thirty seconds and release, take a few seconds of and release and paintings away

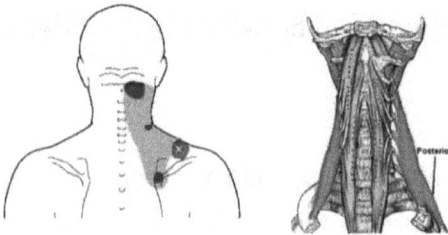

through the areas of anxiety and tenderness.

9. Infraspinatus

Description:

This is a thick triangular muscle springing up out of the internal border and the posterior floor of the shoulder blade. It runs in the path of and inserts into the rear a part of the upper arm.

Function:

It is absolutely taken into consideration one among severa muscle agencies which assist to stabilize the pinnacle arm into the shoulder joint.

Symptoms:

Pain within the outer and upper arm and frequently a sensation of getting a frozen shoulder can rise up.

Trigger Point Therapy:

The motive aspect(s) here are positioned at the shoulder blade and the very excellent way to acquire there, in case you are walking on yourself, then acquire spherical with the alternative hand and hold close the pinnacle of your shoulder at the identical time as searching for to squeeze the again part of your shoulder blade.

Now there may be no specific reason issue, rather you want to enjoy round and search for areas of anxiety. If you may get a helper that will help you with this, then all the higher. The use of a rub down ball or some other hardball is all once more useful right here, whereby you vicinity the ball between the once more of your shoulder blade and a wall and really press again against the wall, preserve for some seconds, release and repeat and then waft from side to side and up and down across the region of the shoulder blade till a brilliant diploma of launch is completed.

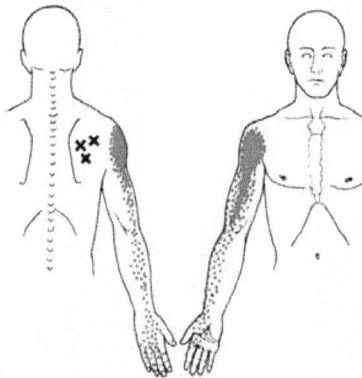

10. Deltoid.

Description:

The deltoid muscle businesses are 3 muscular tissues which join the shoulder to the body and the better arm. They can be cut up into anterior, medial and posterior (the the the front, center and rear).

Function:

Each one works at carrying out some of movement in that unique arc of movement, each developing the arm up, shifting it out to the side or pulling it decrease lower lower back in a rowing movement.

Symptoms:

Atypically shoulder pain stiffens and frozen shoulder commonly is in simplest one plane of motion.

Chapter 15: Glutes And Legs

eleven.Gluteus Minimus

Description:

There are three glutei muscle groups (muscular tissues of the lowest) and this one is the smallest. It runs alongside the pelvis and it originates from the top outer rim of the pelvis and runs downwards to insert into the the the the front outer top ground of the leg.

Function:

This muscle will growth the legs and aids internal rotation of the leg.

Symptoms:

While a small muscle the gluteus minimus can motive quite a few issues and is often tough to become aware of.

It results in ache in the decrease returned, bottom rear thigh and calf. Also it could mimic sciatica pain. And can regularly result in pain radiating out to exclusive trigger elements together with, hamstrings, quadriceps, tensor fascia latae, peroneal and gastrocnemius muscle groups.

Trigger Point Therapy:

There are severa cause elements in this region, the precept ones been posterior gluteus minimus motive, that is in the rear part of the muscle, and the lateral gluteus minimus cause, which lies among the outer rim of the pelvic bone and the hip joint, approximately thirds of the manner up.

The lateral factors can be determined within the anterior fibers (component of the lowest) and are vertically aligned a few inches above the hip joint. So the very excellent way to treat this region is to grab your hip among your thumb, center and forefingers after which squeeze until you can experience the cause point set off, you may furthermore use a massage ball or foam roller if you like.

As for the posterior motive factors, they lie within the posterior fibers which lie in a radial sample, which follows the hip crest arc, but which might be located approximately severa inches under it. In order to locate the ones elements, try to clutch your glute (backside muscle) and sense spherical near the hip joint until you find out an area of tenderness.

Tension inside the glutes, if often hidden, and could require a reasonably rigorous method to each locate and then launch the tension. Do not be afraid to in truth placed pressure on those elements, as no matter the reality that a chunk painful it will result in plenty of remedy to leg, backside and decrease decrease once more signs and symptoms.

Also decrease again pain can often follow due to an imbalance of the glutes (the glutes aren't firing, therefore, they will be no longer sporting the weight) which overloads the lower back, so if you are having decrease lower again issues and ache within the glute location, make a component of working on decrease decrease lower back trigger factors further to glute elements.

12.Adductor longus

Description:

This is a triangular muscle which extends from the pubic bone and runs downwards and outwards to insert into the center zero.33 of the internal aspect of the thigh bone.

Function:

This muscle permits to boost the pinnacle leg and is wanted for abduction of the leg (bringing the leg inwards and throughout the midline of the frame).

Symptoms:

There are cause factors proper right here with the primary one inflicting ache inside the muscle itself and the second one resulting in ache in the the the the front of the hip joint, down the internal if the thigh simply above the knee. This pain can be disturbing and might frequently mimic hip pain.

Trigger Point Therapy:

Start through the use of locating the save you of the pelvic bone inside the crotch place and then skip your hand forward some inches onto your thigh, you need to revel in a sensitive vicinity that is the second reason factor and the number one reason factor is ready   inches better, so in fact elevate your hand up with the

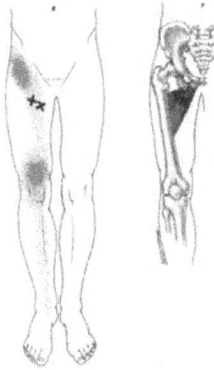

aid of spherical inches and you can find out the primary purpose detail.

 13.Vastus medialis

Description:

This muscle lies on the inner issue of the thigh. It originates close to the pelvis and extends to certainly beyond the kneecap, in which this muscle bulges in the case of those who do quite a few leg wearing activities, this muscle is also referred to as the knee flexor.

Function:

It facilitates to straighten the knee and stabilize the joint. If you ever use a leg extension tool then that is the principle muscle at art work.

Symptoms:

Pain in the kneecap and often ache which feels as though it is radiating out of the knee, moreover a pain within the inner thigh.

Trigger Point Therapy:

The reason factor proper proper right here is just above the bony pinnacle part of the knee. Just preceding to the kneecap itself is a bony outcrop, in reality previous to this is the purpose aspect. It might be very clean to artwork this detail via thumb strain.

Chapter 16: Arms & Hands

sixteen.Supinator

Description:

This muscle runs from the decrease outer aspect of the pinnacle arm down towards the the the front higher problem of the decrease arm.

Function:

This muscle rotates the lower arm outwards, as a way to turn the palm inwards.

Symptoms:

Pain above the elbow and down the outer component of the forearm. It can also radiate ache right right down to the decrease again of the hand above the index finger.

Trigger Point Therapy:

The trigger factor is inside the lower arm virtually beneath the internal elbow crease at the top part of the inner aspect of the forearm, see diagram.

17.Extensor carpil radialis

Description:

This arises from the outer element of the elbow and runs all the way all of the way all the way down to the lowest of the third and second arms.

Function:

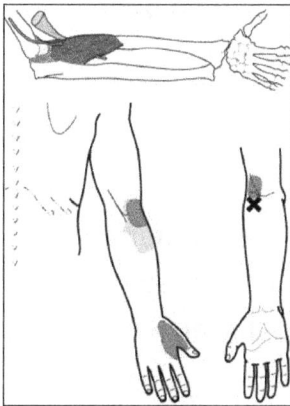

The extension and inwards bending of the wrist.

Symptoms:

Pain above the elbow joint and on the lower returned of the hand. Sometimes entails stiffness and shortage of mobility within the elbow.

Trigger Point Therapy:

This factor is on the anterior issue of the forearm severa inches down from the elbow joint. So it's at the opportunity facet of the forearm to the supinator. So virtually observe the top the the front factor of your forearm, popping out of your elbow joint, and press around until you find a sensitive issue.

18.Middle finger extensor

Description:

This originates at the outer detail of the elbow, shifting downwards, through four tendons, into the lowest of the fingers.

Function:

It enables make bigger the palms, mainly, the

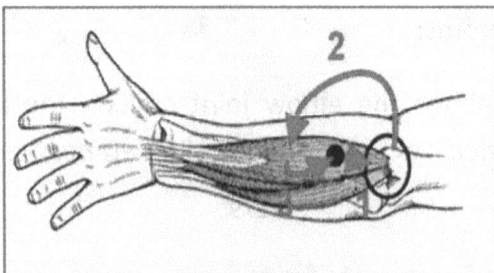

second one and the 0.33.

Symptoms:

Pain in the decrease returned of the hand and down the lower arm. This is frequently an aching ache and often there may be problem in transferring the wrist and palms.

Trigger Point Therapy:

This point is at the lateral thing (thing) of the forearm approximately inches from the elbow joint. Simply have a experience round until feeling a touchy issue and then operating in urgent and relieving the anxiety built up there.

 19.First interosseous

Description:

This muscle runs from the inner, top floor of the bone at the base of the thumb and runs to the aspect of the index finger.

Function:

It helps to bend the index finger and pulls it over towards the thumb while the thumb is open.

Symptoms:

Pain and stiffness in the palm and on the back of the hand specifically near the thumb and the index finger.

Trigger Point Therapy:

This factor is clearly easy to discover. Simply stretch out your thumb and your hands in order that your thumb is pulling far from your forefinger. What results is a triangular shape of flesh which lies among the forefinger and the

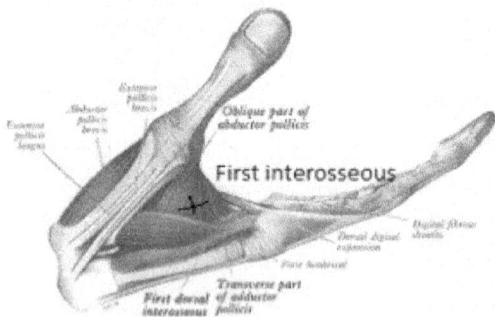

thumb. Simply press all through the midpoint of this fleshy triangle and you can feel the factor.

This is also a famous acupuncture/acupressure component and is called Large Intestine four (LI 4) and it's additionally wonderful for running on expelling bacterial infections from the top. So in case you start getting a head bloodless then pressurize this point for consolation.

20.Abductor pollicis

Description:

This muscle runs from the bottom of the second and zero.33 carpal bones (the forefinger and middle finger) and it inserts into the internal thing at the lowest of the thumb.

Function:

This draws the thumb and fingers together and is the number one muscle to help the thumb bend.

Symptoms:

Pain and stiffness of the thumb specifically inside the outer detail at the lowest of the thumb.

Trigger Point Therapy:

This cause factor is largely in the palm of the hand within the fleshy factor near the thumb, absolutely test the diagram. If you experience round there you'll resultseasily experience a sensitive factor. Simply press and launch it with the thumb of your one of a kind hand.

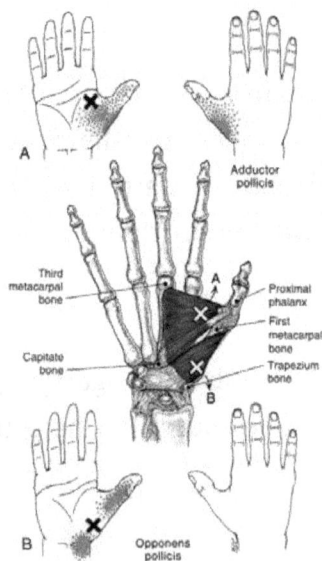

www.ingramcontent.com/pod-product-compliance
Lightning Source LLC
Chambersburg PA
CBHW062140020426
42335CB00013B/1274